EMERGENCY ROOM

EMERGENCY ROOM

Randall Sword, M.D.

Charles Scribner's Sons • New York

The patients and physicians described in this book are composites and the setting is fictitious. But the events could have happened in any of the seven thousand hospitals in the United States.

Copyright © 1982 Randall Sword

Library of Congress Cataloging in Publication Data

Sword, Randall.
  Emergency room.

  Includes index.
  1. Hospitals — Emergency service. 2. Hospitals — United States — Emergency service. 3. Sword, Randall. 4. Emergency physicians — United States — Biography. I. Title.
  RA975.5.E5S88   616'.025'0924 [B]   81-21385
  ISBN 0-684-17271-2   AACR2

This book published simultaneously in the United States of America and in Canada—
Copyright under the Berne Convention.

All rights reserved. No part of this book may be reproduced in any form without the permission of Charles Scribner's Sons.

1 3 5 7 9 11 13 15 17 19 F/C 20 18 16 14 12 10 8 6 4 2

Printed in the United States of America.

For all the nurses, clerks, technicians, paramedics, and doctors who are in the trenches twenty-four hours a day, seven days a week, waiting through the cold, lonely nights for the sick, the injured, and the neglected. These medical personnel have elevated the emergency room from its "converted storeroom" beginnings to its present status as the newest and fastest-growing specialty recognized by the American Medical Association. This is their story.

Acknowledgments

Special thanks go to Janet Keller Tegland, without whose editing help this book would never have gotten into print. Thanks also to Richard O. Sword and Robert F. Scott for their countless suggestions, criticisms, and their encouragement. My fine typist was Joan Durham.

Contents

Preface   xi

1. Coming of Age   1
2. Diagnose, Stabilize, Move On   5
3. Blue Monday   12
4. Cardiac Countdown   32
5. Always Look Twice   54
6. Tell Me Where It Hurts   79
7. Bystander Be Ready   104
8. A True Pandora's Box   120
9. Out, Up, or Down   149
10. No Humans Involved   167
11. Rape—the Invisible Crime   187
12. Diatribes and Digressions   202

Epilogue   215
Glossary   217
Index   219

Preface

THE EMERGENCY ROOM doors swung open.

"Doc! You gotta come!"

I looked up to see one of the cooks from the cafeteria.

"I was walking out to the parking lot just now when this car drives up, dumps a guy out like he's a sack of potatoes, and takes off. I ran over to see if I could help him. I don't even think he's breathing!"

I dropped the chart I was working on and ran outside, shouting for one of the emergency technicians to follow. The man was lying face down in the gutter, his long blond hair spattered with mud. A gold earring in his left earlobe glinted dully.

"Get him on a gurney!" I shouted.

We wheeled him into the emergency room on a dead run. There was no empty bed, so we steered him into one of the cubicles where a woman patient was waiting; we threw back the curtains, pushed her bed against another where a rape victim was vomiting.

"Get the crash cart!" I shouted. "And a number-eight endotracheal tube. We'll hook him up to the EKG." I put the tube down his trachea so we could breathe for him. "Okay, now secure that tube and let's bag-breathe him." The inhalation therapist took over.

I looked up at the scope to see a slow but regular heartbeat. In depressant-drug overdoses, which I knew this case was, the breathing stops first. Then the heart slows and stops, just thirty to ninety seconds later. We were running out of time.

I glanced at the nurse. "Do you have an IV going?"

"His veins are all scarred with needle marks." Her voice was shrill with tension. "I can't get in."

"How are his pupils?"

"Pinpoint," said the technician.

"Give him an ampule of Narcan!"

"I can't! I can't get in!"

I seized the syringe, lifted up the man's tongue, and plunged the needle deep into the tissue underneath, where a rich network of veins lies, giving him the medicine sublingually. This is where heart patients let their nitroglycerin tablets dissolve when they get chest pain.

At least half the patients suffering from drug overdose come out of it fighting, and this one certainly did. Within a minute, after gagging, struggling to breathe, and trying to sit up he started swinging and grabbing at his endotracheal tube. If it hadn't been for the quick reaction of the inhalation therapist who had been breathing for him, he would have pulled the tube out and damaged his vocal cords. His skin, which just seconds ago had had the gray pallor of a sick seagull, was now regaining its color—"pinking up," as we call it. Watching him was almost like watching somebody being born again.

The nurse smiled at me in relief. "What does it feel like to be an instant deity?" she asked softly.

I didn't have time then to reply or think about what she had said, but later, in one of the rare quiet moments on my shift, I thought about the times when emergency medicine (EM; or emergency room—ER) physicians must seem almost like deities to critically ill or injured patients. And I thought about the antithesis of such moments, when everything an emergency physician does and everything he knows doesn't help.

I decided it was time to portray the whole picture of what an EM physician does in a busy hospital emergency room: how he ricochets from brink-of-life events such as cardiac arrests, drug overdoses, or gunshot wounds to the opposite extreme—upset stomachs, headaches, stubbed toes. I hope here to let the reader know what it's like to live with the knowledge that a decision one is forced to make within a few seconds can mean the difference between life and death; what it's like to be the doctor in the emergency room.

1
Coming of Age

IF I WERE TO ASK you to name the fastest-growing medical specialty in America today, would you answer cardiology? pediatrics? immunology? Many are surprised to learn that one of the fastest-growing specialties is *emergency medicine*. In 1978, hospital emergency rooms handled more than 100 million cases, a number that is rising at the rate of 10 percent per year.

If you find this difficult to believe, you may be remembering emergency rooms as they existed in the not-too-distant past when the average hospital emergency room was the last place the sick or injured wanted to go. They knew that when they got there—even if they were in a critical state—they might have to wait as long as thirty or forty minutes for a doctor to arrive. And they knew that the doctor was likely to be a sleepy-eyed intern, an exhausted resident, a harried and impatient staff physician who had reluctantly left a private patient, or a moonlighter who worked in the emergency room because he couldn't get a job anywhere else, because that's how hospitals used to staff their emergency rooms.

Fortunately, all that changed in the past ten to fifteen years, as emergency medicine gained acceptance as an important healthcare specialty.

When I began this book, I realized that the years marking the growth of EM marked significant periods of growth in my own life as well. In 1966, for example, when emergency medicine was just beginning as a specialty, I was twenty-four, winding up a two-year tour of duty with the Peace Corps and trying to get into medical school. Six years earlier I had graduated from high school in Springfield, Pennsylvania, a small town near Philadelphia, without having distinguished myself in any particular way except for a lot of *A*'s in my science courses. I then went to the Philadelphia College of Textiles and Science in Germantown for a bachelor's degree in chemistry and dyeing, but I discovered that I wasn't at all certain I wanted to spend my life working with colors and textiles.

At that time the newly formed Peace Corps was a dream John F. Kennedy had made reality, in an era when helping your fellow man seemed more viable than it has at any time since.

Inspired to do my share, I joined and, together with a fair-sized group of similarly motivated young men and women, entered a six-months' training program on the UCLA campus. I was given room and board and a dollar a day while I studied the culture and language of Ethiopia, the country I had been assigned to. As part of my studies, I read about the diseases endemic to the area where I was going. Delving into diseases like malaria, hepatitis, and smallpox totally absorbed me. During my two years in Ethiopia, I discovered that the people whose company I most enjoyed were the young doctors just out of medical school who were also serving with the Peace Corps.

That was in 1966—the same year the National Highway Safety Act was passed, authorizing the Department of Transportation to set up new guidelines for emergency medical services. Until that time, most ambulance services had been run by funeral homes and staffed by poorly trained personnel. The ambulances themselves were usually equipped with only a stretcher and an oxygen tank. Under the Highway Safety Act, an eighty-one-hour course on the fundamentals of emergency care was designed to train emergency medical technicians. A graduate of this course was designated an EMT-I. A decade after the program's inception, 147,000 persons had received this training. By 1976, EMT-1's constituted the majority of ambulance attendants in the United States.

Emergency medicine took another step forward in 1968, when the American College of Emergency Physicians was founded, establishing the practice of emergency medicine as a specialization in its own right.

At that time I was entering medical school at the University of New Mexico. I had completed two years of graduate study in biochemistry—which was what it took to convince the dean of the medical school that I really wanted to become a doctor.

Two years after I entered medical school, the first physician residency program in emergency medicine was started, at the University of Cincinnati. Now there are over fifty-six hospitals with residencies in emergency medicine.

After I got my M.D. degree in 1972, I served as an intern at the U.S. Army's Gorgas Hospital in the Panama Canal Zone, where I had to spend every third night in the emergency room (ER). The interns at Gorgas literally ran the emergency room. We asked the residents for advice when we needed it, but that didn't happen too often, because when we weren't running the ER we were rotating between stints in general surgery, general medicine, obstetrics and gynecology, and pediatrics. Looking back, I realize I couldn't have had better preparation for becoming an emergency medicine physician.

While I was serving my internship in the Canal Zone, the Mobile Intensive Care Unit (MICU) was being introduced in selected cities in the United States and paramedics were making their first appearance on the scene of medical emergencies. Having MICUs meant that for the first time much sophisticated hospital technology could be brought to a victim in a home or factory or on the street.

At the end of my internship, I returned to New Mexico to work off my debt to the Public Health Service. I was assigned to practice medicine among the Pueblo Indians. Two pueblos, with a total population of eleven hundred, were placed under my care. Much like a general practitioner, I took care of runny noses, sore throats, sprained limbs. If anything more serious occurred, I drove the patient to an Albuquerque hospital.

It wasn't long before I realized that that was where I wanted to practice medicine: in a hospital. So after a year with the Pueblo

Indians, I left New Mexico and became an EM physician in a busy city emergency room.

Two years later, the American Board of Emergency Medicine was established, and two years after that, in March 1980, the first nationwide written and oral examinations were given to establish competency in the new specialty of emergency medicine. Either five years' experience or two years of residency with twelve thousand hours in an emergency room are required before a doctor can take the exams. Passing them certifies that the applicant is qualified to recognize, evaluate, and treat acute illness or injury—that the applicant is qualified as a specialist in emergency medicine.

Because of these requirements, emergency medicine isn't as accessible to the physician just out of medical school as it once was. Previously, almost any doctor could work in an emergency room. No longer. Now the black sheep of the medical profession has come of age. And so—having practiced eight years as an emergency medicine physician, and thriving on every moment of it—had I.

2

Diagnose, Stabilize, Move On

THE DRAMATIC IMPROVEMENT that took place in one decade in the practice of emergency medicine evolved in response to hundreds of thousands of medical emergencies each year. A great need still exists because accidents are the leading cause of death of persons between the ages of one and thirty-seven, and the fourth leading cause of death at all ages.

The 5,000 annual deaths from poisoning, drowning, and drug overdoses could be substantially diminished if immediate emergency care were available.

From 5 percent to 20 percent of the 700,000 deaths resulting annually from heart disease could be prevented if a comprehensive emergency medical system were available throughout this country.

The number of specialists practicing medicine in the United States is increasing, but the number of general practitioners is decreasing. It has become increasingly difficult to establish an ongoing relationship with a general practitioner, and many people who would once have gone to their family doctor for a medical emergency will now instead go to the emergency room of the nearest hospital.

Even patients who have their own physicians will often go directly to an emergency room. They know hospitals are better equipped than doctors' offices, and the emergency room is staffed with a physician twenty-four hours a day. There they won't have to make an appointment, or suddenly discover that their doctor is at a medical meeting or on vacation. And many patients have discovered that their Blue Cross or Blue Shield medical insurance will cover all treatment received in a hospital emergency room, but only partially cover treatment received in a doctor's office.

In addition, physicians in private practice often use the emergency room as an alternate method of caring for patients who need immediate attention. When their own offices are overloaded with patients, or when they are in surgery, attending meetings, or for some other reason unable to attend to such patients, they can refer them to an emergency room, knowing they will receive prompt care.

It is therefore not surprising that the American Hospital Association's figures show that our community hospitals ring up more than 100 million outpatient visits each year, and that the number is constantly increasing.

At least 23,000 of those patients will pass through the emergency room where I work. Some will be brought in by paramedics, some by their families, and some—the majority—will walk in. What's wrong with all these people? In most cases, sprains and strains, cuts and abrasions, sore throats and runny noses, headaches and abdominal cramps, high neck pain and low back pain, infections, dog bites, cat scratches, nose bleeds. These are the garden-variety complaints that constitute 90 percent of emergency medicine. Then there is the other 10 percent: heart attacks, pulmonary embolisms, auto accidents, drug overdoses, strokes, drownings, knife cuts, snake bites, gunshot wounds—the life-or-death-and-make-it-fast-Doc-because-you've-got-ten-seconds-to-decide-what-to-do cases.

Monday through Friday, the busiest time is from four in the afternoon to eleven at night. Sometimes there is a noontime rush that coincides with the lunch hour. On weekends we go full blast from high noon until three o'clock in the morning. There's always somebody waiting to be seen on weekends.

But holidays are the worst. Holidays can bring on my I'm-all-alone-in-the-Snake-Pit syndrome. That's what I call the times when I am under the most pressure, when all around me are sick or hurt people—and I'm the only doctor there. At those times I'm haunted by the specter of examining a boy who is vomiting and has diarrhea and diagnosing intestinal flu when it's actually appendicitis; or examining a young woman with anxiety and shortness of breath and diagnosing hysteria when it turns out to be a pulmonary embolus; or examining a middle-aged man with mild upper abdominal pain and nausea and diagnosing indigestion that turns out to be a heart attack.

There are always two nurses on duty, and one technician and one clerk-of-the-day. But there's only one doctor.

My area in the hospital is called the doctor's room. It's an eight-by-twenty space that contains a bathroom and a shower, a desk, a cot, and the monitor with oscilloscope (called the biocom) on which I receive and respond to paramedic radio calls. Ideally, the paramedic (also known as an EMT-II) will accurately assess a given patient's condition, relay that information by two-way radio to me, and receive instructions from me as to what, if any, medical procedures should be performed before transporting the patient to the hospital. That's the way it works on television, but the reality—as I will point out in chapters to come—is often different.

When a patient comes to my emergency room, it's my job to diagnose and stabilize that patient, and then, if he or she needs continuing care, to contact a physician who will provide it and under whose aegis the patient will then be admitted to the hospital.

Sometimes patients have their own physicians whom I can call, but if they don't, I have to find a doctor for them—which isn't always easy.

The present era is one of specialization. There are twenty-three "official" specialties, ones that are recognized by the American Medical Association, and approximately twenty others that are not yet formally recognized. The more specialized the medical profession becomes, the more one specialty is insulated from another. This has its drawbacks, because a given specialist tends to look at one particular kind of tree and lose track of the existence of any other kind, let alone ever cast an eye at the entire forest. But it also has its advantages: a specialist tends to master all the fine points of his or her specialty and can keep abreast of all the latest developments in it. The EM physician, who is constantly referring patients to other doctors, must be cognizant of these specialties.

When I have to contact a specialist for one of my patients, I use a call list of doctors who are on the hospital staff. All active staff members are required to take their turn in the "Snake Pit," which is what they affectionately call the emergency room. Each of the fourteen departments inside the hospital has a separate rotation list. On a given list, a doctor's name will usually come up only once or twice a month. As soon as the list is compiled, it is mailed to each doctor, who is also reminded by phone the day before he or she is on call.

On paper, the call schedule looks good. In reality, it often breaks down. Sometimes physicians forget they're on the schedule and leave town; sometimes they don't carry their beepers and can't be contacted if they are away from a phone; sometimes they're busy at another hospital. Almost every day—and invariably every night—I have some problem with the call schedule. Theoretically, however, once a physician's name is on the list, it's up to that physician to either accept my calls or see that someone else will. But patient care remains the responsibility of the EM doctor until another physician can be contacted to assume responsibility.

And while the EM physician may be the one who brings a patient through a severe medical crisis, it often happens that the EM doctor will never even see that patient again. That's the nature of the job. Diagnose. Stabilize. Move on.

Sometimes I think being an emergency medicine physician is a lot like being a news photographer. Each patient I see is a distinct entity, having no connection to the next. Snap. Click. Move on.

And for many people, their contact with me constitutes their first hospital experience. What happens to them inside the emergency room may well determine their attitude toward future hospital care. So no matter what shape I'm in, I try to make the experience as agreeable as possible.

I may come to a patient emotionally drained and in a state of near exhaustion, having spent the previous hour trying to save a life. If I failed, I'll be asking myself the perpetual questions that plague all of us who work in this business: "Could I have tried something else?" "Did I do the best possible job?" "Could someone else have saved him?" What I really need is time to sit and sift through the events, to try to put them in the right perspective. In short, I need time to unwind. But there's a patient waiting to be seen, and I have to be able to walk into a room smiling—because patients who come to hospital emergency rooms are interested in just one thing: their own condition. They're not interested in the fact that minutes ago I pronounced a man dead and have just come from informing his family.

Sometimes I want to release it all and share my troubles and self-doubts with them. I can't—it wouldn't be ethical or appropriate. And so I smile and say, "Hello, I'm Dr. Sword. How can I help you?"

If they're there for a valid medical emergency, they claim my full attention and I stop thinking about what happened before. But if they're there for a nonemergency reason, like a sore throat or a headache, my thoughts may drift. And if I'm really tired, I'll be tempted to say something like, "Why the hell did you wait until three in the morning to come in if you've been sick for the whole week?"

I don't say things like that, because I know what the answer would be: "I couldn't sleep, Doc. And I didn't want to bother my own doctor at this hour." *I* know 3 A.M. is a much lonelier time than 4 P.M. And I also know that sometimes it's easier to bother a stranger. Which is what I am to them, and will remain.

I don't get emotionally involved with my patients on a long-term basis. In fact, most of the time—after they leave the emergency room—I never see them again. I suppose it sounds odd sometimes when I describe to friends or acquaintances a particularly interesting or dramatic case, and they ask, "Well, what happened to the patient?" and I have to say, "I don't know." But that's inherent in the nature of emergency medicine. When 23,000 patients a year pass through the bailiwick where you work, you don't have the time or the emotional capacity to find out what happens to all, or even most of them. In fact, were I inclined on occasion to say to myself, "I think I'll go up to Cardiac Care and see how my heart attack patient from yesterday is doing," I'd be stopped before I got out the door—with "Dr. Sword, we have a cut finger on Bed 8, a stab wound on Bed 6, and a swallowed penny on Bed 2." But I knew that when I went into emergency medicine—and I accepted it.

Compensating for the fact that I'm not able to establish long-term relationships with my patients is the ongoing sense of adventure I get from emergency medicine. I never know what I'm going to see next. I can go from an overanxious mother with a basically healthy child to the mangled victim of a hit-and-run accident. I read somewhere that emergency medicine is like a kind of yoga exercise: relaxation alternating with total concentration. I couldn't agree more.

One of the reasons I went into emergency medicine is that I don't like to deal with chronic problems like diabetes, hypertension, arthritis, obesity, and cancer. Often the specialists who deal with these problems aren't able to cure the patients, so they just treat the symptoms and try to make life easier for their patients. But I like to see a problem, solve it, and then move on to something else.

And still another reason I went into emergency medicine is that I haven't the expertise, the inclination, or the aptitude to manage an office. The hospital manages my office; it takes care of the billing, the insurance forms, the government forms, the accounting problems, and the myriad personnel problems. Coping with these would only distract me from why I'm in medicine: to practice it.

During my twelve-hour shift, I give medicine everything I've got. When it's Snake Pit time, I wrestle with the snakes. And at the end of my shift, I simply pick up my coat and go home.

Often, after I've been working the night shift, I'll arrive home anxious for some sleep just when everybody else in my house is getting ready to start their day. It's always hard for me to tell my fourteen-year-old son, Tod, that if he wants to listen to his stereo during the day he's going to have to wear earphones; and no, he can't have his friends over unless he gags them as they walk in the door. And it's hard to tell my preschool-aged daughters "Good night, Daddy's going to bed now," when it's 8 A.M. and they want me to go to the beach and build sand castles. And it's hardest of all to know my wife Sandra has to walk around on tiptoe most of the day telling our three normal, rambunctious children to be quiet.

But there are advantages, too. At least I know that once I drive away from the hospital, that's it. I will never be called at home in the middle of the night (or day) and asked to come in to see a patient.

In the pages that follow, I'm going to try to give you an idea of what it's like to be an EM physician. I'm going to take you into the Snake Pit with me. I'm going to walk you through nine of the emergency medicine classifications in which I am expected to be an instant expert. Along the way, I'll also share some of the funny things that happen that help all of us get through the bad times.

If you're a pre-med student, and you're thinking about becoming an EM physician, this book will give you some idea of the gamut you'll have to cover. If you're a paramedic, or a young person thinking about becoming a paramedic, you'll learn what happens on the receiving end of the biocom. And if you're a future patient, well, you might like to know what will happen to you in the emergency room. And why.

3

Blue Monday

SUPPOSE THAT YOU, or someone you care about, or a stranger that you encounter on the street is experiencing chest pain. How can you tell if it's a heart attack?

I wish I could give you a sure-fire formula, but I can't. The evaluation of acute chest pain is one of the most frequent and critical problems encountered by an emergency room physician. The doctor must rapidly and accurately distinguish between the more grave conditions that carry the prognosis of sudden death and the many less serious causes of chest pain. To make things more difficult, there isn't much relationship between the severity of the chest pain and the gravity of its cause.

Chest-wall syndromes are common causes of chest pain that require differentiation from cardiac pain. Localized inflammation of the upper central ribs or cartilages, nerve root compression, and muscle cramping may all give the appearance of a heart attack. And rib fractures, common in alcoholics who don't recall experiencing any trauma because they were drunk when it happened, may be mistaken for heart attacks.

Often there is little correlation between where in the chest the pain is located and the source of the pain. Because the esophagus lies right behind the heart and the stomach lies underneath the heart, inflammation of the esophagus, stomach, or pancreas—or even gallbladder spasms—may all simulate a heart attack.

This means, of course, that the person with chest pain can't really tell whether the pain is of gastrointestinal or cardiac origin. But there are certain signs that can be recognized. Usually pain of gastrointestinal origin has a burning character, is relieved by antacid therapy, and is related to posture (that is, the pain increases when the patient lies down). If the chest pain does not present these characteristics, the person suffering the pain should immediately see a doctor.

Unfortunately, people experiencing what may be a major medical crisis often diminish their chances for survival by trying to answer all the "what-ifs" before they seek help: "What if I can't afford medical treatment?" "What if my doctor will think this is just a minor problem and be irritated with me for bothering him?" "What if my family thinks it's just my nerves again?" "What if I can't continue to work?" "What if I can't take care of my family?" Plagued by such doubts, many people take no action at all. Consequently, of the more than 650,000 people who die of heart disease each year, about 350,000 of these die outside a hospital, usually within two hours after the beginning of symptoms. This is why heart disease is the number-one medical emergency in the United States today.

Harry Denise was the victim of such an emergency, as was Cora Adams.

It was a Monday morning when I met Harry and Cora. Blue Monday.

Pulling into the hospital's parking lot, I glanced up at the big red-and-white Emergency sign. Despite the early morning fog, it stood out starkly.

I was beginning the 7 A.M. to 7 P.M. day shift. I work the day shift for five days straight, have five days off, and then work the night shift (7 P.M. to 7 A.M.) for five days.

As I entered the hospital, I saw the night crew leaving. Dr. Walker was grim-faced with exhaustion. "Hello, Randall," he said gloomily. "Nothing left over for you. We'll see you tonight." And he walked out to his car.

"Have a good rest," I murmured, and wondered, God, do *I* look that bad after a night shift? Hell, I decided, I probably look worse. Even so, sometimes I still have a small boy's dream-cloaked idea of doctoring ... of people dressed in immaculate white running around saving lives. One memory also keeps me going: At the age of sixteen I watched my own father die in an oxygen tent, and would have given anything to be able to save him.

I went on into the EM physician's room and changed into the faded green surgical scrub suit, over which I put a long white coat. I glanced into the main treatment area. In it there are seven curtain-screened cubicles, each containing a mobile white-sheeted stretcher. Overhead cabinets are filled with liter-sized bottles of fluids for IVs, with catheters, depressors, cotton swabs, syringes, test tubes—all the paraphernalia for emergency treatment. Beyond the main treatment area, separated from it by a wide arch, is the two-bed critical care area.

Located behind the glass partition of the nurse's station are the staff members who work with me. There's Gloria—dark haired, about twenty-five, a damned good nurse with a tendency to be highly emotional. Shirley is a petite blond with robin's-egg-blue eyes and an infectious laugh; she hasn't been an emergency room nurse very long, so she's always asking questions and trying to learn—which I like. Mark is a lean, edgy youth who works as an emergency medical technician for $3.85 an hour to pay for his karate lessons. Alice, the admitting clerk, is a woman in her mid-fifties who is an ardent believer in silver linings. Her favorite three words are "is doing fine": "Your husband is doing fine." "Your wife is doing fine." "Your child is doing fine." Once she told a woman, "Your husband is doing fine," just as I was starting to fill out his death chart. Her job is not an easy one. The admitting clerk is the patient's initial contact with the hospital. While reassuring the patient that something will be done as quickly as possible, the clerk has to get all the necessary information: if they have insurance, where they live and work, their Social-Security number. Patients often assume that admitting clerks have some medical training, but they don't. All they have to know is how to type and what the admitting procedures are. Probably because the frequent crisis situations are so stressful, most clerks last only a few months or a year. But Alice has been at Memorial for sixteen years, telling people they're doing fine.

My first patient that blue Monday was a Mrs. Cook, who had

sliced open her index finger with a steak knife while washing dishes. I was sewing up her finger in the main treatment area when Alice called out that she had a man with chest pain in the admitting room. As Gloria brought him through the sliding glass doors in a wheelchair and whisked him to the critical care area, I saw that he was a stout, ruddy-faced man with a worried expression, holding a clenched fist to his chest. A thin, birdlike woman carrying a small paper bag tried to follow him through the emergency room doors, but Alice called after her, "Mrs. Denise, the doctor and the nurses will take care of your husband now. I have some papers and forms for you to fill out."

Mrs. Denise held up the brown paper bag. "But I have his medicines here."

"I'll give them to the doctor," Alice countered firmly.

"Couldn't I please just stay with my husband?"

"I'm sorry. There are other patients. Visitors only add to the congestion. The doctor will come out and talk to you later. If you will just fill out this form . . . I'm sure your husband will be fine."

The sliding doors closed, separating the woman from her husband.

As I sewed up Mrs. Cook's finger, I heard Gloria help the man out of the wheelchair and onto the narrow bed, then snap up the side rails to enclose him. Mark went in to begin pasting the four one-inch electrode leads on Mr. Denise's chest in preparation for the cardiac monitor. One lead would be placed near each shoulder and one below each nipple.

"Are you taking any medicines?" I heard Gloria ask.

"Yes. My wife brought them in a paper bag."

"What are they?"

"I don't know. My wife brought them. Can't she come in?"

"Did you take any medicine before coming in here?"

"I took two nitros under my tongue."

"Did that make the pain go away?"

"Not like it usually does."

I knew Gloria would turn on the cardiac monitor after Mark finished attaching the wires. Gloria later told me that at first the scope looked as if his heart were in fibrillation (beating irregularly at four hundred to five hundred times per minute—which would result in death in a few minutes). Alarmed, she glanced at his chest and noticed that one of the leads had come loose. When she reattached it, the scope changed to a nice regular beat.

Mark, I knew, would be turning on the oxygen meter and adjusting the volume flow to six liters per minute. He would then wind the long blue-green oxygen tube around the patient's head and fasten it under his nose, where it would make a hissing sound.

Mr. Denise must have been startled; most patients are.

"It's only oxygen—to help you breathe," I heard Mark say reassuringly.

"Are you short of breath now?" Gloria asked.

"No."

"Does the pain go down your arms?"

"My left arm did feel heavy and a little numb, now that you mention it."

"Do you feel sick?"

"I did earlier. I felt like I was going to vomit, but I didn't."

"Blood pressure 140 over 90 . . . respirations 18 . . . and pulse 110," Mark read off Mr. Denise's vital signs.

Every fifteen minutes, Gloria will automatically record the patient's data on the flow sheet she is beginning. She will continue to record these, the medications that are given, and any changes in the patient's status. In addition, a heart-rhythm paper tracing strip is run from the monitor, then clipped to Gloria's notes with the time it was taken indicated. A constant record is thus kept for each patient from the moment he arrives in the critical care area, and it becomes part of the permanent hospital record.

Alice passed through the main treatment room on her way to the critical care area. She was holding a brown paper bag and a legal-size chart. I heard her say, "Gloria, here's Mr. Denise's medicine." And then: "Mr. Denise, we need your signature for your 'consent to treat' and to pay all bills not covered by your insurance."

"Where do I sign?"

"There at the bottom. Have you ever been a patient here before?"

"No."

"All right. I'll get the rest of the information from your wife. Now I'm going to place this yellow arm band around your wrist for identification, and then I'll leave you with your nurse. I'm sure you're going to be just fine."

"Mark," Gloria said, "would you call the EKG technician to come and do an electrocardiogram? I'm sure we'll want one."

"Sure."

Then Gloria came briskly through the wide arch to the main treatment area where I was finishing Mrs. Cook's hand. "We have a forty-seven-year-old man with chest pain," she said. "Do you want me to start an IV?"

"I heard his vital signs," I said. "How is he looking?"

"Like he's had one."

"Go ahead with the IV then. I'll be right there."

She nodded and left the cubicle. A minute later, I heard her say, "Mr. Denise, the doctor said we have to start an IV." And I knew she was brandishing a two-inch needle.

"A what?" he exclaimed.

"We need to insert a needle into one of the veins in your arm so we can give you medication rapidly should the need arise."

The needles come in various sizes and lengths. Most are one and a half to six inches long, with a plastic catheter fitted snugly over the end and an exposed metal tip. After the needle enters the vein, the metal tip is pulled back, leaving the flexible plastic catheter in place. The catheter is threaded very gently up the vein for an inch or so. The other end is connected to plastic tubing that is connected to a bottle hung on a bracket over the patient.

It's not an easy procedure. Many veins are "blown" when the tip breaks through their thin wall and the blood leaks out, causing ballooning under the skin. But with an IV correctly in place, we have instant direct access to the forty thousand miles of blood vessels that traverse the body.

Giving medicine by mouth rather than through an IV is usually impractical in emergency situations for several reasons. First, it takes time for the medicine to dissolve. Often an hour goes by before adequate blood concentrations are reached. Second, many medicines are digested by the stomach acids and rendered useless. And last, the patient may be too sick to take medicine orally. He may even be unconscious at the time he needs medicine the most.

Medicines given intramuscularly by needle bypass these problems, and generally take effect faster than those given by mouth. But medicine injected into the muscle still has to dissolve and filter into the bloodstream before it can be distributed throughout the body. In addition, it is often absorbed irregularly and incompletely, so we cannot depend on getting a prescribed concentration at a given time.

Medicine given intravenously is available throughout the body within seconds. But the very speed with which it circulates can create risks. Most medicines that may safely be given by mouth can be given intravenously only with great caution, and some medicine cannot be given intravenously at all. Drug reactions are much more likely to occur with an IV and can be fatal.

At last I finished Mrs. Cook's finger and went to the critical care area.

"Mr. Denise, I'm Dr. Sword. I understand you've been having chest pain. Can you tell me about it?"

"Well, I was finishing up some weekend painting on the back porch. I was bending over washing my brushes when I felt like I had a muscle cramp in my chest. I straightened up, but it seemed to get worse. I put a nitro under my tongue, but it didn't have the usual effect, so I took another one. When I began to sweat and feel sick, my wife brought me here."

"How long did the pain last?"

"I don't know, maybe thirty to forty minutes. I wasn't watching the clock."

"Has the pain eased up any?"

"Some, but it's still there. Feels like someone sitting on my chest."

"Gloria, give Mr. Denise six milligrams of morphine sulfate IV. Mr. Denise, did the pain seem to travel anyplace—like to your neck, jaw, or arms?"

"Well, as I was telling the nurse, my left arm felt heavy and then numb."

"Did you vomit or feel nauseated?"

"When I straightened up with the brushes I thought I was going to get sick, but I didn't."

"Any shortness of breath—difficulty in breathing?"

"I couldn't seem to catch my breath for a while there."

"Did you sweat?"

"At first I just felt hot, then the sweat poured out of me, like I stuck my head in a bucket, dripping from my nose. My wife had to get me a towel to dry off. Look, am I having a heart attack?"

"Let me ask a few more questions, finish examining you, get an EKG; then I'll be in a better position to answer you."

"Did you call my doctor?"

"After I fully evaluate you, I'll call your doctor. There's no use calling him now. The first thing he'll ask me is how your EKG looks. Now, since you've been taking nitros, you must have had this chest pain before. What sort of problems have you had with your heart?"

"Dr. Taylor gave me the pills and told me to put one under my tongue when I got chest pain, and if two didn't help, to come directly to the emergency room."

"How often do you get pain in your chest?"

"Oh . . . not too often."

"When was the last time?"

"A few days ago. I was walking up the little hill near my house to get the evening paper. I got the same sort of pain or pressure, but it stopped as soon as I rested. Just part of getting old, I guess, huh, Doc?"

"How many times have you had pain in your chest during the past few weeks?"

"Three or four, I guess. . . . I really don't keep track. It usually only lasts a minute or two and I feel fine afterwards."

"So exercise or exertion seems to set off these attacks and they ease off rapidly if you rest."

"Yes."

"How would you describe the pain? Sharp? Dull? Pressure? Burning? Constant?"

"Constant. Aching pain, like someone sitting on my chest."

"Is this pain different from previous times?"

"More intense, lasting longer. And no matter what I did, the pain remained. I tried belching, thinking it might be gas. I took some Alka-Seltzer and lay down. Then I broke out in a heavy sweat and had trouble breathing. It felt like someone was choking me."

At that point the EKG technician arrived, and I had him start.

"What do you think?" Gloria asked as I walked over to the nurses' station to write on Mr. Denise's chart. The charts are hung in two rows on hooks on a large clipboard, with the bed numbers in big red numerals on the cover of each.

"Well, he sure gives a textbook history: sudden onset of left-sided pressurelike pain lasting thirty to forty minutes, radiating down his left arm with associated symptoms of nausea, sweating, and shortness of breath. Then he gives me a classical history of angina: short episodes of chest pain with exertion, stopping shortly after ceasing the activity. He could have written the book."

Angina pectoris is chest pain of cardiac origin and is at one end of the spectrum of heart pain. It's caused by the heart muscle's not getting enough oxygen. No permanent damage is done, and a person can have an unlimited number of these attacks. They are usually associated with exertion—when the heart has to pump hard and fast, thereby increasing its own need for oxygen. When the demand for oxygen outruns the supply, pain begins; the demand must be slowed down so the supply can catch up.

At the other end of the cardiac spectrum the oxygen is reduced to a point where the heart muscle is damaged or permanently destroyed. Medically this is called an infarction or a coronary; it is more commonly known as a heart attack.

There are many points between these two extremes, and not every case is as clear-cut as Mr. Denise's. Angina does not necessarily lead to or precede a coronary.

Alice stuck her head into the nurses' station. "Do you want to talk to Mrs. Denise? She's awfully anxious to know what's going on."

"I'll wait until I've had a chance to look at the EKG, then I'll have that much more to tell her. It should only be a few more minutes now."

By the time I'd finished writing on Mr. Denise's chart, the EKG was ready. It showed a normal pattern. All normal electrical activity of the heart starts from a small bundle of muscle fibers and nerves, called the sinoatrial mode, or pacemaker. The activity travels in a wave spread along well-defined pathways, causing the muscles of the heart to contract in a rhythmic fashion. It's a little like a rock thrown into a pond which causes waves to spread and touch all the shores at a set interval of rhythm. This electrical pattern can be picked up, magnified, and recorded on a strip of paper known as an electrocardiogram (ECG or EKG). Any change in the pattern will show up with a characteristic altered tracing.

When I had finished reading Mr. Denise's EKG, I told Alice to tell Mrs. Denise to come in. The fragile-looking woman I had glimpsed earlier came through the sliding doors.

"Hello, Mrs. Denise. I'm Dr. Sword."

"Is my husband having a heart attack, Doctor?"

"Let's go where your husband is resting so I can talk to both of you."

Mrs. Denise was obviously startled when she saw her husband lying in a bed with railings up and with four wires coming from his chest, a tube from his nose, and a bottle with a long tube running into his arm. But she managed a weak, "Hi, honey. How do you feel?"

He tried to smile and reassure her. "Better."

She turned to me. "Is he going to be all right?"

"Your husband's EKG is essentially normal right now," I said. "However, the characteristic pattern that we see in a heart attack can take hours or even days to develop. Many physicians admit a patient with a past history of chest pain to the cardiac care unit regardless of what the EKG shows. I feel this is the best course for your husband."

"Thank you, Doctor. We'll do that, then."

"Is that really necessary?" Mr. Denise interposed. "I do feel better now."

"You don't have to listen to him, Doctor," Mrs. Denise said.

"Well, he is a grown man and he does have the right to refuse . . . I mean, I'm not going to tie him to the bed. I do advise admission, however. It's better to be on the conservative side and put him in the Cardiac Care Unit than to have him go home now and develop a fatal heart attack that could have been prevented.

"You see, Mr. Denise, the most dangerous time in a heart attack is the first twenty-four hours, and the most dangerous part of that is the first two hours. That's when irregularities of the heartbeat are most likely to occur. If you're here in the hospital, they can be corrected by drugs, often with life-saving results."

"Did you call my doctor?" he asked.

"Not yet. I wanted to look at your EKG and have a chance to talk to you. We'll call your doctor now."

"Well, can't you tell me straight off—without all this mishmash of EKGs, CCUs, and two-hour business—did I or didn't I have a heart attack?"

I shook my head. "I can't answer you with absolute certainty. If you stay, we'll take EKGs and blood tests every day, and that will help us answer that question. It's kind of like making a chart on a blank piece of graph paper. The first point doesn't mean as much as two points, which can indicate that the graph is going up or down. With three points, you have a curve and may see a trend developing."

"Dr. Sword, excuse me, but Dr. Taylor is on extension 595," Alice called to me.

When I spoke with Mr. Denise's doctor, I told him I thought Mr. Denise had suffered a probable myocardial infarction, a heart attack, and should be admitted to the cardiac care unit. Dr. Taylor agreed, saying he would come to the hospital when he had finished with his office patients. I wrote the CCU orders, started the blood work, and ordered a chest X-ray so that it would be ready when he arrived.

I had scarcely finished doing this when Shirley asked me to come to the main treatment area.

"What's up?" I asked.

She was blushing. "It's this little boy," she said. "His penis was crushed by a toilet seat."

I winced at the thought.

Shirley led the way into one of the curtained cubicles, where a stocky, muscular man with black hair stood beside a small boy who held himself and stared straight ahead while tears streamed down his cheeks.

"What happened?" I asked.

"It's like I was telling the nurse here. He was urinating and the seat fell down on his penis. He's been holding it ever since. Won't let anyone look at it."

"How old is he?"

"He'll be three in August."

"What's his name?"

"Pedro."

"Pedro, I'm a doctor. Let me see what happened to you."

"No!" Pedro wouldn't even look at me.

"Pedro," the father said, "let the doctor look at you."

"No!"

"Pedro, I'm not going to hurt you. All I want to do is look."

The "no" this time was softer, and a little less sure.

With the help of Shirley and the boy's father, I slowly pried the child's fingers, one by one, away from his penis. He screamed the entire time. But it wasn't nearly as bad as I had imagined. It was a little swollen, and black and blue around the tip. But the skin wasn't broken, so I didn't have to suture it, and the small testicles weren't injured.

I said to the father, "Normally, I'd suggest using ice to keep the swelling down. But I don't think he'll let you. Anyway, it's just a bruise in a bad spot. He'll be sore for a few days. You may want to watch him urinate for the next few times to help him get over his fear, and to check for signs of bleeding. I doubt there will be any, but if there is, he should be checked again."

"Right, Doc. Thanks."

As I left the main treatment area, Alice told me that Mr. Denise's bed was ready in the cardiac care unit. I told Gloria and Mark to take him there as soon as he was hooked up to the portable monitor, and I headed for the coffee urn. I was just lifting a cup to my lips when the bell in the doctor's room sounded, indicating a paramedic run. I put down my coffee cup and hurried in to answer the call.

"This is City Rescue Two, come in Memorial. This is City Rescue Two, can you hear us, Memorial?"

"This is Memorial Hospital base station. I can hear you loud and clear."

"Okay, Memorial. We have a sixty-eight-year-old woman with shortness of breath and some chest pain. This developed suddenly thirty minutes ago when her daughter called us. She is sweating heavily, anxious looking, with poor color. Her vital signs are: blood pressure 210 over 120; pulse 130; respirations 32 and shallow. Did you copy?"

"Ten-four, Rescue Two. Hook her up to the monitor and send me a strip of lead two when you're ready."

"Ten-four. Here's lead two coming at you."

The paramedics use the same four standard electrodes that we use in the hospital: one at each shoulder and one below each nipple. The recording is radio-transmitted so I can read out the rhythm from the oscilloscope. This procedure does not replace the twelve-lead standard EKG that is taken in the hospital to diagnose a heart attack; it is only used to rapidly transmit information about an emergency patient to a distant doctor.

"Okay, Rescue Two, this is Memorial. That's enough of lead two. She looks as if she's in a rapid sinus rhythm. Start an IV of D_5W and put her on oxygen."

D_5W is 5-percent dextrose (sugar) in water. The paramedic can start an IV and give drugs only under the direction of a doctor at the base station. No diagnosing is done in the field; if the situation is very urgent, as in the case of Mrs. Adams, treatment can begin in the field, but usually the patient is transported to the base station for definitive care.

I asked, "Do her lungs sound wet?"

"No, Memorial. Her primary problem is difficulty in breathing, but not much chest pain per se."

"Okay, Rescue Two. What is the patient's name?"

"Mrs. Cora Adams. She's been at Memorial before."

"Bring her in Code Three, Rescue Two." Code 3 means red lights flashing and sirens wailing.

"Will do, Memorial. Our ETA is five to ten minutes."

I glanced at the clock. "Ten-four, Rescue Two. This is Memorial Hospital clearing the frequency."

I asked Alice to get me Cora Adams's chart, thinking—as I

waited—that I would probably never get over the feeling that I'm practicing medicine in a fishbowl whenever I take a paramedic call. In any given region, radio frequencies are shared with other base-station hospitals. Thus, a doctor's assessment of information and the appropriateness of his responses are open to instant peer review by every physician (not to mention nurse, paramedic, and amateur-radio fan) tuning in to the same frequency. In addition, all paramedic runs are taped and then gone over in periodic tape reviews. No less litigation conscious than most doctors, I have spent a few sleepless nights.

Alice brought me Mrs. Adams's chart. It was almost two inches thick! I scanned it quickly. It said that on her most recent admission, which was her ninth, she suffered a pulmonary embolism. I wondered if she'd had another one.

A pulmonary embolus is usually a clot of blood broken off in a large vein in the legs or pelvic area. It can also be fat or other foreign material. These float up and get stuck in the filtering system of the lungs, causing a blockage of blood through that part of the lungs.

Sirens screaming, the paramedics arrived with Mrs. Adams. Shirley was ready and waiting. "Put her on bed one," she ordered, "and we'll hook her up to our monitor. Mark, could you hold the IV bottle? Mrs. Adams, you *must* keep your arm straight, or else you'll lose that IV and we'll have to start another one."

Until the nurses get the patient settled, I customarily stand at the foot of the patient's bed, either giving orders or just observing and acting as a coordinator. I have found that if I get involved in starting an IV or pumping on someone's chest during a resuscitation, I can lose my perspective. It's up to me to view the patient as a whole and keep everyone else on target.

Turning to the paramedics, I asked, "How is she doing?"

"About the same as in the field," was the answer. "Her blood pressure came down some and the oxygen helped her breathe easier. Her color looks better, too."

Most paramedics take pride in and feel comfortable with their role. Once in a great while a paramedic may decide to substitute his judgment and authority for the physician's, and then things can go terribly wrong. Fortunately, this is the exception rather than the rule. Once the paramedics have delivered the patient to the ER personnel their responsibility is over. Sometimes they'll stay to see how a patient is doing, to chat or have a cup of our dreadful coffee, but they are actually free to be called out on another run. Paramedics take a special training course (it varies from state to state), but they are not doctors or nurses and their function is limited to rescuing patients, stabilizing them, and transporting them to the hospital.

"Mrs. Adams, I'm Dr. Sword. Can you tell me what happened?"

Mrs. Adams didn't look good. She was in obvious respiratory distress.

"I suddenly felt short of breath," she began, taking in three rapid, shallow breaths. "I felt like someone was choking me." She stopped again to catch her breath. "Some pain came here." She circled her left breast with her right hand. "I started coughing." Gasping again, she put her hand to her throat. "I even coughed some blood up."

"How long has your left leg been swollen and red like that?"

Still gasping, she responded, "I've had arthritis in that knee for years now. Dr. Powers has been treating me for it." She rested for a moment, then began again. "The leg has doubled in size and has become oh, so sore this past week." Another rest. "The redness has been there since yesterday. I've spent the past week in bed. I can't stand to put any weight on my leg."

"Well, Mrs. Adams, we'll get an EKG, some X-rays of your chest, and some blood from your arm."

I turned to Alice. "You can get most of the information from her old chart. I don't think she's going to be able to answer any more questions now."

Then I told Mark to call Pulmonary Therapy and tell them we needed a set of blood gasses stat (meaning as quickly as is humanly possible). Measuring the blood gasses (the oxygen and carbon dioxide in the blood) gives us an indication of how well a patient is exchanging air as he breathes. Part of the magic of the human body is that the lungs have an effective surface area about the size of a tennis court. On this surface, oxygen from the air is absorbed into the red blood cells. It is also on this surface that the waste product, carbon dioxide, is extracted out of the blood into the lungs. The exchange takes place in less than one second, and it's a delicate procedure whose balance is easily disrupted. An embolus, or blood clot, can throw off the measurement of the oxygen and carbon-dioxide content of the blood by having a damming-up effect, causing blood to bypass that particular area where the exchange takes place. The larger the clot, or the more clots there are, the less surface area remains for the gas exchange to take place.

If the set of blood gases obtained indicates the possible presence of a clot, a lung scan can be useful in confirming it. Radioactive material of a specified size is injected into the bloodstream through a vein. This material travels throughout the body but is caught only in the lungs' filtering system. The clot will show up on the scan as a lung area that is not radioactive, because blood is bypassing it and not flowing through it. However, there are other conditions, such as pneumonia, abscesses, or tumors, that may also cause a decrease of blood flowing to a given area of the lung, so a lung scan in itself does not prove the existence of a clot—though in conjunction with symptoms it tends to confirm it.

If surgery is being contemplated to remove the clot, and it's necessary to know the clot's exact location, angiography is done. A small catheter is inserted into a large vein in the groin and slid up two to three feet into the right side of the heart. Dye is injected, and very rapid multiple X-rays are taken. The dye will outline the clot. An angiogram can be hazardous, and it's only done to facilitate the surgery.

The only alternative to surgery is to maintain the patient on anticlotting drugs like heparin or Coumadin, which stop extensions of the clot and give the body a chance to dissolve it.

I asked Alice to call Mrs. Adams's doctor.

A few minutes later she told me that Dr. Powers was not available, but that another doctor was taking his calls. I told her to call him, wondering if there was going to be any difficulty. I can't admit patients into the hospital myself. My contract states that I will limit my practice solely to the emergency room. Sometimes a doctor covering for another physician is reluctant to admit that doctor's patients to the hospital—especially critical care cases—since he doesn't want to become involved.

Mrs. Adams certainly needed to be admitted.

"I couldn't agree more," the doctor said when Alice got him for me on the line. "Unfortunately, I'm no longer on the staff at Memorial. You can transfer her to my hospital, or perhaps your backup medical-staff man on call today would admit her and cover until Dr. Powers returns."

I thanked him, hung up, and asked Alice who our medical backup was today.

"Dr. Silver."

"Damn," I said. "I hate to call him for anything, much less a sick patient. He should have retired years ago. Probably the only journals he reads now are *Medical Economics* and *Business Week*." I shook my head. "Go ahead and give him a call anyway."

We were stuck. We have to call the backup doctor first if the patient needs to be admitted and doesn't have her own private doctor.

Within a few minutes, Alice had him on the line.

"Dr. Silver," I said, "we have a little problem here. One of Dr. Powers's patients is here in the emergency room. Dr. Powers is out of town for several days, and another doctor is covering for him. However, this doctor isn't on our staff, so he has no admitting privileges. He suggested that you manage the patient until Dr. Powers comes back."

Dr. Silver quickly countered, "How about transferring her to that doctor's hospital?"

"Well, this is a sixty-eight-year-old woman with a probable pulmonary embolus, and if you saw her, you wouldn't want to transfer her across the room, much less across town. Besides, she lives nearby and she's been here before, so all her records are here."

There was a beat of silence, during which I pictured Dr. Silver marshaling all the reasons why he shouldn't be the one to admit Mrs. Adams. I was right.

"I can understand your position, Dr. Sword. I've worked in emergency rooms myself. But I don't like to be dumped on, either.

Dr. Powers should have known better than to have a doctor who isn't on our staff take his calls. It's his problem."

It was a good thing he couldn't see my face, because he wouldn't have liked my expression. "Dr. Silver, Dr. Powers cannot be reached. I have a gravely ill woman here fighting for her life. It's my neck if she dies before she gets to another hospital. She needs to be admitted to our intensive care unit. *You* are our medical backup today for the emergency room."

"I'm sorry, Dr. Sword. I have an office full of patients who also need me—and have appointments. My first responsibility is to them, and I intend to get back to them now."

Grimly I asked, "Can you suggest another doctor?"

"I don't know the case. It's better that you try to find someone."

In a voice made of icicles, I said, "Thank you very much for your help," and hung up before I could hear his response.

If a patient who doesn't have a doctor needs to be admitted and is too sick to be transferred to the county hospital, it is the responsibility of the doctor on call to assume care of that patient. If there is a disagreement between the on-call physician and the emergency room physician as to whether or not a patient should be transferred, the on-call physician must come to the hospital and assume responsibility, in writing, for the transfer of the patient. Usually, the on-call physician accepts the judgment of the ER physician and this doesn't become necessary.

Admitting privileges can be suspended or revoked for actions such as Dr. Silver's. By rights, I should have called the chief of service or chief of staff. But making trouble can work against an emergency room doctor. And my immediate concern was my patient.

"Try Dr. Booth," I finally said to Alice. "He's new on staff and might need the business."

She reached him quickly. New doctors are usually easy to reach.

"Dr. Booth," I said, "we have a disposition problem here: a critically ill woman with no admitting doctor. Her own physician is out of town, the back-up doctor he uses is not on staff, and the on-call doctor is too busy. Can you help us out?"

"Sure, I'll come down and take her off your hands."

I was grinning with relief when I hung up the phone.

"Admit Mrs. Adams to Dr. Booth," I said to Alice, "and transfer her upstairs to the intensive care unit *stat!*"

I cast my eye hopefully toward the coffee urn, but Gloria came out of the main treatment room and blocked it from my view. "Dr. Sword, now that you're off the phone, we have a little boy waiting with an earache."

Behind the pale green curtain, I found a small boy holding his hand to his right ear while sitting on the lap of a very beautiful woman, whom I asked, "How long has he had an earache?"

"When I left for work, he was fine," the woman replied in a husky voice that matched her face. "But when I came home from work, the baby-sitter said he had been holding his ear and crying. I took his temperature. He has no fever, and he ate all of his lunch, so he can't be feeling all that bad."

"Has he complained of a sore throat or runny nose?"

"Do you have any of those things, Jeffrey?" she asked him.

Jeffrey looked mournfully from his mother to me and back again without answering. As I removed him from his mother's arms, tears welled up in his brown eyes. When I placed him on his side with his right ear facing up, he didn't say a word or make a sound.

The canal of the ear is about one inch long and is shaped like a lazy S. To see down to the silvery drum, pull the ear back, out, and up—to straighten out the canal. The drum itself is pearly white and looks like an oval, paper-thin membrane—hardly broader than an eraser on the end of a pencil. Earwax, or cerumen, is secreted and formed by glands located only in the outer two-thirds of the canal. Earwax serves a purpose, catching dirt and keeping insects (which find the pungent odor and taste of the wax disagreeable) out of the canal. Using a cotton swab to clean the ear only serves to pack the wax closer to the drum. The cotton swab, with its big bulky end, cannot get behind the wax and pull it out. The wax itself offers no impediment to sound. Only when the wax is pushed against the drum itself, keeping it from vibrating, does it interfere with hearing. The old saying, "Put nothing smaller than your elbow in your ear," is good advice.

I peered into Jeffrey's ear and I smiled. "He's got a bean in his ear!"

His mother's eyes widened in surprise. Then she started to laugh. "Better check the other ear. Maybe he's got popcorn in that one."

Taking a pair of alligator forceps, I pulled the bean out easily.

Jeffrey left me with a smile—holding on to his mother's hand.

"We'll stop for ice cream," I heard her say. "What flavor do you want?"

"Strawberry," Jeffrey replied.

I wished she'd asked me, I thought as I left the cubicle.

Gloria was waiting outside.

"Dr. Sword, we have a patient who . . ."

4

Cardiac Countdown

EVERY TIME I COME ON DUTY, every time I walk into my eight-by-twenty-foot room, I wonder how many times the biocom will ring during this shift, how many times the mundane *ding dong* will call me to respond to a possibly life-and-death situation. When the paramedics call me, what I think and say can make the difference between someone's living and dying. Note that I said "what I think and say," not "what I do." I can *do* nothing.

I can think of only one other occupation in which anything like this happens. Even there it occurs rarely, and more often on television than in real life. The situation: when the traffic controller in an air control tower must verbally and from a great distance give instructions to some poor stewardess or passenger on how to fly the plane, because something has happened to the pilot.

Of course paramedics have to know more about medicine than flight attendants or passengers do about flying airplanes. But there is a tremendous variation in current training programs for paramedics. Some programs run a hundred hours; some run fourteen hundred hours. As a result there are great variations in the skill levels of the ten thousand paramedics presently in the field. EM physicians sometimes have reason to feel that working with paramedics is like practicing medicine in no-man's land.

When I take a paramedic's call on the biocom, I am expected to diagnose a patient I cannot see, feel, or touch—and this runs contrary to all of my professional training. I must rely on the judgment of a stranger whose ability level I do not know; and even if I knew that the paramedic's skill level was high, I wouldn't know his or her panic level or tolerance level for dealing with a critically injured person. I may have to instruct this stranger to initiate a complicated medical procedure inside a mangled automobile amid hysterical bystanders and impatient police officers, knowing all the while that I am just as responsible for those injured people whom I cannot see as I am for those I treat in person. In fact, I may very well be busy treating someone inside the hospital when the biocom summons me. But I know there has to be some degree of urgency for the paramedics to have called.

One of the things I most frequently get called about is severe chest pain.

When I picked up the biocom on one particular night, the sound of the siren was audible in the background. I could hear the tension in the paramedic's voice as he said, "This is County Rescue Sixty-five. Come in, Memorial Hospital." And I suspected we were in for a Code Blue.

"Memorial, we have an elderly male here who is in full cardiac arrest. We were transporting him to County Hospital for treatment for alcoholism when he collapsed. Since you're closer than County, we're coming to your place."

"This is Memorial, Rescue Sixty-five. Do you have an IV line in?"

"That's negative."

"Do you have him hooked up to the monitor? Can you send me a rhythm strip of lead two?"

"We haven't had time to put the leads on yet. We were only transporting him to County, since he couldn't drive himself."

"Okay, Rescue Sixty-five. Continue doing CPR and bring him in. What is your ETA?"

"We're turning off Highway One now, onto Rose Avenue. Our estimated time of arrival is three to four minutes."

Three to four minutes! I shouted at the rest of the staff, "Let's move! We have a Code Blue coming in."

Every time a cardiopulmonary resuscitation, or Code Blue, is called, butterflies start performing a ballet in my stomach.

As an emergency medicine physician, I am required to respond to all Code Blues that occur inside the hospital. I don't have time to be nervous; I just start running to wherever it's happening.

But when the paramedics are bringing one in, although I have plenty of things to do, I also—unfortunately—have time to be nervous while I'm doing them. I usually clear the area of all other patients in order to protect the privacy of the person needing CPR. I check the crash cart to see that it's equipped with the medicine, various sizes of tubing, needles, mask, oxygen tank, and fluids that we use. While I'm checking the cart the nurses pull the headboard off the bed so that we can work around the patient on all sides. The other beds are pushed away, and a one-inch-thick, two-by-three-foot wooden board is placed on the CPR bed to provide a hard surface against which we can "pump" the patient's chest.

While I wait, I also go over the *ABCD*'s inside my head: *A* is for airway, *B* for breathing, *C* for circulation, and *D* for definitive therapy.

No matter how many times I go through all this, the wait always seems longer than it actually is. I once read that soldiers in combat experience this same sense of time elongation. Men involved in sudden, sharp skirmishes will swear that the battle went on for hours, when actually the action was over in ten or fifteen minutes.

As I went through the *ABCD*'s for what seemed like the five hundredth time, I began to hear the sirens coming closer and seconds later I saw the red lights reflecting off our windows.

"Here they are!" someone yelled.

The electric doors flew back. Two attendants pushed and pulled the stretcher through the open doorway, while another attendant pumped continuously on the patient's chest. He was performing external cardiac compression, counting out loud: "One-two-three-four-five and breathe, one-two-three-four-five and breathe," while still another attendant was bent over the man on the stretcher, performing mouth-to-mouth resuscitation on him at the end of each count of five.

This kind of external cardiac compression is performed in cases of cardiac arrest when there is no pulse and no breathing and the victim is unconscious, with a deathly appearance. The rescuer uses the heel of one hand, covered with the other hand, on the lower half of the victim's chest. Positioning his shoulders directly over the victim's chest, the rescuer keeps his arms straight so he can lean the weight of his body forward onto the victim to compress the sternum, or breastplate, about one and a half to two inches. The compressions must be regular, smooth, and uninterrupted. The heel of the hand doesn't leave the chest. The heart is actually squeezed between the sternum and the backbone. The compression is released once per second during a count of five to allow the sternum and ribs to recoil to a normal position, with the second rescuer inflating the victim's lungs at the end of every five seconds.

The cardiac compression technique used on children is slightly different. Only one hand is used, the sternum is compressed only three-fourths to one and a half inches, and it is repeated eighty times a minute, rather than sixty.

With infants, only the tips of the index and middle fingers are used to compress the sternum one-half to three-fourths of an inch, and the rate is at least one hundred per minute.

Cardiac compression has certain hazards. If you push too hard, you may fracture a rib or two. In fact, this is almost unavoidable in elderly people because their rib cages are so stiff. Believe me, it's chilling to hear and feel ribs cracking at the beginning of CPR. But if you press too lightly you won't be effective. Also, if you compress too low you may lacerate the liver—and if you compress too high you'll force blood back into the heart instead of out of it into the rest of the body.

Before external cardiac compression can be performed, the mouth of the patient must be cleared of food, blood, vomitus, or mucus, and the airway must be cleared. This can be done quickly and without any equipment or help from another person. With the victim lying on his or her back, the rescuer—in order to tilt the victim's head as far back as possible—places one hand under the victim's neck and the other hand on the forehead. This maneuver extends the neck and lifts the tongue away from the back of the throat. Because the tongue is a muscle, it will relax in an unconscious person and fall back against the throat. No one actually swallows their own tongue; but in a relaxed position against the back of the throat, the tongue can block the passage of air. To prevent this from happening, the victim's head must be maintained in a backward position at all times, or a soft plastic airway must be inserted into the mouth. Sometimes simply tilting the victim's head back is all that is necessary to restore spontaneous breathing.

However, if spontaneous breathing doesn't begin after the mouth and airway are cleared, the rescuer must start mouth-to-mouth resuscitation. Keeping one hand behind the victim's neck, the rescuer continues to maintain the victim's head in a maximum backward tilt. The rescuer then pinches the victim's nostrils together with the thumb and index finger of the other hand while using the palm of that hand to exert continuing pressure on the forehead. Then he opens his mouth widely, takes a deep breath, makes a tight seal around the victim's mouth with his own mouth, and blows into the victim's mouth. He then removes his mouth and allows the victim to exhale passively. This cycle is repeated once every five seconds for as long as the victim is unable to breathe independently.

When performing artificial ventilation on a child, the rescuer should cover both the mouth and nose of the child with his mouth and use smaller breaths to inflate the lungs once every three seconds.

When performing artificial ventilation on an infant, the rescuers should use only a puff of air in his cheeks. Anything stronger than that might blow out an infant's lungs. And nobody should attempt CPR who has not taken a course under supervision and practiced on mannikins.

As I looked at my CPR victim being wheeled inside, I asked one of the attendants manipulating the stretcher if he had any information in addition to what was relayed to me on the biocom.

"Not much," he replied. "His name is John Gootee. He's

about sixty-three. When we picked him up, his wife said he'd been hitting the bottle pretty heavily for the past two or three weeks. She said she wanted him 'dried out.'"

"Did she mention any medications he's on? Any previous heart problems?"

"No. She would hardly speak to us. She just wanted him out of the house. But I've rolled on him before, so I know he has a long medical history. He's been in and out of County Hospital like a boomerang for years."

I shook my head. "Well, this may be your last roll on him. He looks terrible. His color is already ashen gray." I turned to Alice who was standing by, watching. "You'd better call his wife and get her down here."

While I was talking to the attendant, Gloria and Mark had gotten Mr. Gootee off the stretcher and onto the bed with a back board under him. They had also placed an ambo bag—a compressible rubber bladder with a tight-fitting mask that allows no air to escape—over his mouth. Squeezing an ambo bag with the hand isn't any more effective than breathing directly into someone's mouth, but it's a lot more aesthetic.

Suddenly Gloria shouted, "Dr. Sword, he's vomiting."

"Damn!" I exclaimed. "Roll him over on his side!"

His lungs certainly couldn't function well with his last night's dinner blocking them off. I could see that in order to insure adequate ventilation, and to prevent Mr. Gootee from sucking his own vomitus into his lungs, we were going to have to do an endotracheal intubation. I asked Gloria for an endotracheal tray, on which were various sizes of soft plastic curved tubes. The adult sizes are about eleven inches long and one-half inch in diameter. A balloon cuff is attached to one end of the tube and inflated after insertion, to hold the tube in place; this forms a closed system—air can't leak around it, and oxygen can be delivered under pressure to the lungs. The other end of the tube is left sticking out of the mouth so that it can be connected either to the ambu bag (for hand ventilation) or to the automatic breathing machines. Once I had this tube placed correctly, I could put Mr. Gootee on machines that would exchange air for him, controlling the volume, the number of breaths he took per minute, and the pressure and the percentage of oxygen he received. The machines are even cycled to sigh, because sighing is important—it's nature's way of assuring that we take a deep breath whenever we need one so that we use the outermost parts of our lungs, thereby preventing them from collapsing.

When I first got out of medical school, I dreaded having to intubate a patient. Anything put down the throat, including the endotracheal tube, tends naturally to go through the esophagus and then into the stomach. And blowing air into the stomach is disastrous. Not only does no oxygen get into the lungs (where it is badly needed), but the air will distend the stomach and cause its contents to come back up. As soon as you find out you went down the wrong way and remove the tube from the esophagus, the stomach acid rushes down the trachea into the lungs. Sometimes I would go down the wrong way and blow up the cuff, only to find out I was in the stomach. I would have to deflate the cuff, take out the tube, and try again, angrily regretting the precious minutes I had lost. During my internship, I practiced endotracheal intubation under supervision on surgical patients in the operating room. But even at the end of my internship I still didn't feel I was good enough at this procedure—in which saving a few seconds can mean saving a life. So I practiced on medical-school cadavers. And when people died in the emergency room, I practiced on them as well.

Of course, practicing on cadavers offered ideal conditions. I was all alone, and my cadavers offered no resistance. It's an entirely different matter to intubate a patient in an emergency room, with someone pumping on the patient's chest at the same time I'm trying to see where I'm going with the tube. Now I can usually put a tube into someone's trachea in ten to fifteen seconds—unless I have a patient whose neck is stiffened from arthritis, or one who has a thick bull neck like a prizefighter's, or one whose throat is filled with blood . . . or vomit. Like Mr. Gootee's.

I asked Gloria to help me pull him up a little on the bed so that I could get behind him to open his jaw.

In order to open the jaw, I use an instrument with a lighted handle attached to a six-inch-long curved blade. This instrument will open the jaw and slide over the tongue at the same time.

I rolled Mr. Gootee from his side onto his back, tilted his head backward into the "sniffing position," and opened his jaw. I could see nothing but vomit.

"Give me some suction," I ordered.

On the wall behind me was a long clear-plastic hose connected to a vacuum pump and a trap. The hose is used to suck out blood and vomit from a patient's throat, mouth, and lungs; the trap catches whatever I suck out.

As I pushed the curved blade over Mr. Gootee's tongue to insert the suction hose, he retched again, sending his last night's dinner all over my hand and down my arm.

"Damn! The suction is clogged with spaghetti. Get me a new suction—a bigger one!"

Lifting up on the curved blade, I looked for the epiglottis—the fingernail-sized, rubbery pink bit of tissue in the throat that hangs in a semicircle and normally prevents food and water from getting into the lungs. Then I looked for the vocal cords. Fighting back the impulse to vomit myself as I sucked out stale wine, I further extended his neck to bring his mouth more in line with the trachea. There were the cords. Now, if I could just slip the tube between them ... Done! I was in!

"Inflate the cuff," I said to the inhalation therapist, Greg, who had arrived just moments before. "Then pump him a couple of big breaths so I can listen to his lungs to be sure I haven't put the tube down too far."

If the tube is put below the point where the trachea divides into the right and left main stems, only one lung will be ventilated. This will result in the collapse of the lung that is not being ventilated. Fortunately, I had placed Mr. Gootee's tube at just the right point.

I nodded at Greg. "Secure that airway now with some tape."

Then I asked Shirley, "Do we have an IV line established yet?" I glanced at her as I sponged off my hands and arms, and swabbed at the places where my pants had been stained. I'd have to change as soon as I could find the time.

Shirley was working intently over Mr. Gootee's arm. "I've had the needle in the vein several times," she replied without looking up. "But each time I advance the catheter, the vein blows up. His veins are like tissue paper."

"Don't use a tourniquet," I told her. "Old people's veins are fragile, and a tourniquet can cause too much pressure on them. Try it without."

When the heart isn't pumping, there is no pressure to hold open the veins, so they collapse. Veins that are collapsed are very difficult to get into. But as I mentioned before, it's important to get an intravenous line in place as quickly as possible so drugs can be introduced directly into the bloodstream and distributed throughout the body in seconds. In situations like this, we just don't have the time to give drugs by mouth or intramuscularly.

Watching Shirley struggling over Mr. Gootee's arm, I wondered if I'd have to do a venous cutdown, which involves cutting through the skin, finding a vein, digging it out, and threading a very thin flexible tube up into it—a tube within a tube, so to speak.

As I finished drying my hands, I asked, "How are we coming with that vein now?"

Shirley's eyes as they darted up at me from the patient were a glacial blue. "Just about, *Doctor* Sword."

I snapped, "Look, if you can't get in the vein, tell me, and I'll do a cutdown." The tone of my voice slashed through the room. I could see Shirley was as tense as I was, and I already regretted having raised my voice. It was a definite sign I was losing control, and I fought to regain it. Normally I pride myself on being cool and objective in difficult situations. There are some days when I think I could run a successful CPR on my own mother—but this wasn't one of them.

"Got it!" Shirley announced triumphantly. "Flowing beautifully."

I smiled at her, hoping she was in a forgiving mood. She was, and smiled back.

"Is he hooked up to the monitor?"

She handed me a strip. It looked bad: asystole, which means his heart had no electrical activity.

"Give him two ampules of bicarb through the IV," I told Shirley.

Sodium bicarbonate is given to counteract the acid that rapidly builds up in the body once the heart stops pumping the blood around. "Follow the bicarb with one ampule of adrenalin, and then an ampule of calcium chloride," I continued.

All the time the nurses were carrying out my orders, the attendants were keeping the CPR going: "One-two-three-four-five, breathe . . . One-two-three-four-five, breathe."

I can't stress enough how important teamwork is in CPR. You have to have people who know what they are doing and are good at doing it. My job is to be the coordinator, to stand back and maintain objectivity, being ready to order whatever medicines are needed and watching the entire team—the person pumping on the chest, the person breathing for the victim, the person starting the IV, the person putting on the chest leads for the monitor, the person getting the medicines ready and injecting them when told to inject them, and the person recording on the flow sheet the time and amount as each medicine is given. If I get too involved and start pushing on someone's chest, I can't maintain my command of the whole situation; I can't think of all the drugs, give all the orders, make certain the patient is being well ventilated.

As I said earlier, I'm required to respond to all Code Blues in the hospital. More often than I like to acknowledge, I will run into a room and see a physician pumping up and down on someone's chest. I'll know right then and there that that physician doesn't know what the hell he's doing. Doctors who feel they're effective only if they're doing something with their hands will pump on the patient's chest for a while; then they'll pause to see if the IV is running; then they'll look around for somebody to come and put an endotracheal tube down the patient's throat. They don't want to do it, because the last one they put down was a year ago—and then it took them three tries. They'll pause to look up at the monitor, and then they'll order some more drugs. And all along they'll be shouting the same orders to four or five different people, making everyone else just as nervous as they are.

So no matter how much I may *want* to do something with my own hands, I've learned to stand back and maintain my perspective of the entire situation.

"Look!" Gloria exclaimed. "The monitor is showing some fine fibrillation."

The heart has two phases: the first, systole, occurs when the heart pumps blood out to the rest of the body. In the second, diastole, the heart fills up again with the blood returning to the heart from the body. When the rate of the heartbeat goes above 140 to 160, there just isn't enough time for the heart to fill up. In fibrillation, the heart is beating 300 to 600 times a minute. Different parts of the heart are contracting independently, and the heart itself looks and feels like a quivering ball of worms. The first time I saw and felt a heart in fibrillation was a dog's heart in an experimental laboratory, and it sent chills up my spine.

When the heart is in fibrillation, beating five hundred times per minute, there are many "pacemakers" operating independently to set the beat, instead of the usual one pacemaker, the sinoatrial node. Remember the analogy I used before to explain that the electrical activity of the normal heart is like the ripples made on the water when a stone is cast into a quiet pond? The waves created go out in all directions in a nice, even, rhythmic manner. In fibrillation, to continue the analogy, it's as though hundreds of stones were thrown into the pond all at once from every side. To override all these independent centers of activity, we use defibrillation paddles to deliver a strong electrical current for 1/1000 of a second. This calms the waters again by creating one strong center to wipe out all the competing centers, allowing the heart's natural pacemaker to take over again.

As soon as I saw Mr. Gootee's heart going into fibrillation, I ordered Gloria to get ready to use the defibrillation paddles to shock him with four hundred watts.

She looked around anxiously. "Where's the conduction paste?"

I handed her the tube of paste to smear over the two-inch round silver fibrillation paddles. The paste prevents the skin from being burned when the shock is administered. Gloria placed one paddle to the right of the sternum above the nipple, the other below the nipple on the left side.

"Oxygen off! Stand back!" she ordered.

Zap!!

For a brief second, Mr. Gootee looked as if he were getting up from the table. His back arched and his arms and legs jumped . . . but his face was still a death's mask.

I looked up at the monitor. He was in coarser fibrillation. Instead of beating five hundred to six hundred beats per minute, his heart was beating three hundred to four hundred.

"One-two-three-four-five, breathe . . . One-two-three-four-five, breathe," was still going on in the background as I told Shirley, "Give him a hundred milligrams of lidocaine." Lidocaine is a potent drug used to decrease the excitability of the heart and therefore the tendency for the heart to have multiple pacemakers or electrical centers.

"The lidocaine is in," Shirley announced.

I told Gloria, "Shock him again."

"Stand back!"

Zap!!

Again his back arched, his arms and legs jumped. But his heart continued to fibrillate, and the death mask remained.

The attendants, sweating out their one-two-three-four-five, breathe, looked up at me. I knew they were wondering when I was going to give up.

Avoiding their eyes, I looked down at the man whose life was ebbing away. I checked his pupils. They were still fixed and dilated. I wondered if I should call it off.

The responsibility for stopping a CPR effort lies solely with the doctor in charge. Generally, if the pupils are fixed and dilated, and there is no response to the drugs and shocks after ten to fifteen minutes, I will pronounce a patient dead. But this is an extremely difficult thing for me to do—especially if the patient is an infant or a child. I ask myself, "Do I have the right to pronounce this person dead?" And then, "Should anybody have that right?" I've often kept CPR teams working over a child for as long as four hours, only to have to tell them, finally, to stop; then I go and inform the child's parents that we failed. There are certain situations when we will just "go through the steps"—for the family's sake, so they will know that we did everything that could have been done; or for purely legal reasons, when we're not really expecting much to happen. We know that if elderly people don't respond in the first few minutes, they won't ever.

It's always my personal preference to let people die in dignity rather than prolong the dying process to no purpose. What good does it do to hook someone up to a machine that will breathe for the patient for a few days, or even a few weeks—if the patient is neurologically dead and will die of pneumonia or kidney failure anyway? Even if people are weaned from the breathing machine, few are ever the same afterward. The expense is enormous . . . and I'm not just talking about money; I'm talking about the emotional toll on family members who watch helplessly as their loved one is hooked up to some damn machine. You can see what's going on from their faces. Sometimes, of course, they're wishing, hoping, praying their loved one will get well. But often they can't help wishing, hoping, and praying that it will just end.

The mechanical creation of a limbo state in which a patient is neither alive nor dead seems to me to unnecessarily prolong the agony for everyone, including the doctors and nurses. Sometimes I think if we're going to keep people alive on machines, then we also need machines to run our emotions for us.

Thoughts like these were running through my mind as I watched the team working over Mr. Gootee. Finally I made my decision. One more try, and that would be all.

To Shirley, I said, "Add another ampule of bicarb and another of adrenalin."

To Gloria I said, "Wait thirty seconds, then shock him again."

"Stand back, everybody."

Zap!!

For the third time, Mr. Gootee's back arched up and his legs and arms jumped, and all eyes went to the monitor.

And by damn if we hadn't gotten it: a regular beat.

You could almost hear a cheer go up. As hard and unfeeling as we try to become—because we lose so many of these patients over the years, and we have to be able to live with that—it's always good to save a life, and it always will be.

"Have we got a pressure yet?" I asked Shirley.

"About eighty over forty," she replied.

"Well, we'll have to build up his pressure. Put eight hundred milligrams of dopamine in five hundred cc's of a five-percent sugar solution, and start the drip at thirty drops per minute. Check and see how he's responding to that rate after five minutes. And in the meantime, get a blood-gas study."

As I mentioned before, measuring the oxygen and carbon dioxide in the blood gives us an indication of how well a patient is exchanging air as he breathes. During the past fifteen minutes, while one attendant had been pushing on Mr. Gootee's chest, another had been breathing for him through the endotracheal tube, with 100 percent oxygen. The blood-gas study would tell us how well we had succeeded in ventilating him.

I took another look at his pupils, which a few minutes before had been fixed and dilated. After breathing stops, it takes thirty to forty-five seconds for this to happen, even though brain death takes much longer: four to five minutes. (Infants can survive even longer than that. The younger the brain, the less sensitive to anoxia—deficiency of oxygen—it seems to be.)

Since he was still unconscious, it was impossible to determine whether or not Mr. Gootee had suffered brain death. But after good ventilation, and with his heart going again, his pupils had begun to constrict. It was a good sign.

Gloria asked, "Do you want a Foley catheter in him?"

A Foley catheter is a rubber tube the thickness of a pencil which is inserted into the bladder through the penis. An attached balloon is blown up at the end of the catheter so it won't come back out. Under normal conditions, urine is produced continuously by the kidney and stored in the bladder, and a person will urinate when the bladder is full. But when a patient is unconscious and unable to urinate on command, a Foley catheter hooked up to a urinometer enables us to measure the hourly urine output. Urinary output is the best indicator we have as to whether or not the tissues of the body are receiving an adequate blood supply. If they are not, the body—in order to conserve what blood there is—will preferentially shut off blood to all but the most vital organs, the brain and heart, by narrowing the arterial tubes that transport the blood. This narrowing is called vasoconstriction. The first area that is shut down is the skin, which then becomes cool, clammy, mottled, and takes on a bluish tinge. The next area to be shut down is the digestive tract, and then the kidneys. When this happens, the kidneys will stop producing urine and the body will cease to be able to get rid of its wastes. This is why we want to measure the amount of urine on an hourly basis. A urinary output of one ounce per hour is considered minimal; we like to see four or five ounces per hour in an adult. Anything less is an indicator of shock. (With children, it depends upon their weight.)

I nodded at Gloria, telling her to use a number 18 catheter.

Then I turned to Shirley. "How's his blood pressure doing now?"

"Ninety over fifty-five," she replied.

Which wasn't good.

"Turn up the dopamine drip to fifty drops per minute," I told her. "We've got to get him out of shock."

While urinary output is our best indicator as to whether or not the tissues of the body are receiving an adequate blood supply, another good indicator is blood pressure. If it is very low, the heart is not able to continue to pump blood into all parts of the body, and the patient will go into shock.

Although the term *shock* is used quite generally by newspaper and television reporters, there are actually four distinct types. The most common is hypovolemic shock, which is caused by loss of fluid volume in the body. This can be a loss of blood; or in burn victims, loss of plasma; or in cholera victims, of liquid stool. The heart requires a given volume of fluid in order to be able to pump. If the body loses liquid volume, there will be a decrease in the blood volume coming back to the heart. When the heart senses a lack of fluid, it compensates by beating faster. When it can no longer do this, the blood pressure begins to fall and the patient goes into hypovolemic shock. We treat this condition by administering fluids.

In the second type of shock, cardiogenic shock, giving fluids would only make things worse. Here the primary problem is heart failure. There are already plenty of fluids and an ample supply of blood, but the heart just isn't working well enough to pump, or circulate, the fluids, and eventually the tissues become flooded.

The lung is flooded first, resulting in pulmonary edema, or "wet lung." To treat cardiogenic shock, what is really needed is a new heart, or pump. At the present time most people who go into cardiogenic shock die, and it is to prevent this that there has been so much work done in recent years on artificial hearts, heart valves, and heart implants.

A third type of shock, far less common than either of the above, is neurogenic shock. This type occurs in spinal cord injuries, or complications of anesthesia. It can also be caused by extreme fright. In neurogenic shock, the blood doesn't return to the heart, but pools instead in the peripheral veins and tissues of the body. Fortunately, the condition is usually temporary. It is best treated with fluids and with drugs that cause the blood vessels to constrict. Anaphylactic shock—caused by a reaction to a stimulus such as a bee sting or a penicillin shot—is a sub-type of neurogenic shock.

The cause of the fourth known type of shock, septic shock, is not yet clearly understood. The most common initiating event seems to be the death of bacteria in the bloodstream. These dying bacteria give off poisons, resulting in damage to the tissues and blood vessels, which in turn results in a pooling of blood similar to that in neurogenic shock. These poisons, called toxins, seem to retard the pumping action of the heart. This type of shock usually occurs in the elderly and is difficult to treat, since it is so often complicated by the other problems with which the elderly can be plagued. The treatment is aimed at destroying the toxin-producing bacteria while at the same time keeping up the blood pressure with cardiotonic drugs. Toxic shock syndrome is a newly recognized variation of septic shock.

Shortly after Shirley increased the dopamine drip, Mr. Gootee's pressure went up to 110 over 70. I told her to maintain it at that level and to keep me informed as to his urine output.

Even though his color was better, he still wasn't breathing on his own. I knew he was too unstable to be transferred to County Hospital, where he had been headed. We would have to admit him here and use our backup cardiologist.

Alice had been coming back every few minutes to see how Mr.

Gootee was doing. "Who's our backup in cardiology?" I asked her.

"Dr. Nebulon," she replied.

I told her to give him a call, hoping that I could ease back and relax—at least for a little while. I should have known better. Before she went to call Dr. Nebulon, Alice informed me that while we had all been working on Mr. Gootee, two more patients had come in: a woman who had swallowed her gold dentures, and another, who was raving about a fly in her ear.

There are many phrases that describe how I feel about moments like these: "From the sublime to the ridiculous" is one; "From lions to polecats" is another.

I asked if the woman who had swallowed her dentures was in pain. Alice shook her head. "Actually, she seems to think it's kind of funny."

"Then send her down for an abdominal X-ray," I said. "And I'll go have a look at the . . . fly in the ear."

When I entered the green-curtained cubicle, I saw a thin woman lying on her side with her left hand cupped over her ear. This one certainly didn't think anything was funny. She sat up and looked at me with worried hazel eyes.

"Oh, Doctor, thank goodness you've come. Every time I move, *it* moves. It's driving me crazy."

"How did this . . . uh . . . this fly happen to get in your ear?"

"I was hanging my clothes out to dry, and suddenly it flew right in. I didn't actually see it, but I think it's a fly. It *has* to be a fly. What else could it be?"

I shook my head. I didn't know.

"Oh! It's moving again." She started crying. "Please get it out; I can't stand it."

Gloria had followed me around the curtain, and I told her to get me an otoscope so I could examine the ear.

As I pulled the woman's ear back, out, and up I inserted the end of the otoscope and looked through the magnifying viewer into her ear canal. At first I didn't see much. Then what appeared to be a large piece of wax came into view. But this "piece of wax" had black and grey stripes, was covered with black hair, and as I peered at it, it moved. Startled, I drew back. The thing had apparently flown in and then couldn't turn around in the narrow ear canal to get back out.

"It's in there all right," I announced.

"I *know* it's in there. I told you that. Can't you do something? Give me a shot or something?"

I said, "I'm going to put some mineral oil in your ear. The fly will suffocate and float out." I know insects can only breathe through their shells or skins. And although I had never actually performed such a procedure, it certainly sounded logical.

"You can't do that," she responded.

"Why not?"

"I have a hole in my eardrum, and my ear doctor said *never* to put anything in my ear."

"Hmm," I said.

"Doctor? *Please?*"

A few minutes earlier, I'd been saving a man's life. Now I was doing battle with a common housefly. It seemed to me that if I could be forceful in the first situation, I should be able to master the second.

"Gloria," I said forcefully, "get the alligator forceps."

"What are you going to do?" the woman asked.

"Get hold of the damn thing and pull it out," I said.

Gloria, biting her lips to keep from laughing, handed me the forceps.

"Hold perfectly still," I told the woman.

"It's moving," she whispered tensely. "I can feel it moving."

"Just about . . . no, it keeps going deeper . . . hold still now . . . got it!"

I held the fly out triumphantly for the woman to see. I was glad that it was still wriggling; a live fly made me seem much more heroic than a dead one.

The lady beamed at me. "Oh, thank you, Doctor."

I nodded magnanimously and left, thinking—masterfully— now . . . on to the lady with the dentures in her stomach.

The X-rays were ready. She did indeed have dentures in her stomach. Wondering how she had managed to swallow them, I went to ask her.

She was sitting up on the bed assigned to her, with a bemused expression on her face.

"I'm Dr. Sword," I said. "I've just heard about your problem, Mrs. Kovar."

She looked at me and shook her head. "Oh, Dr. Sword. Sword?"

I nodded.

"I'm so embarrassed. I've had these dentures for years. I'm still not exactly sure what happened, but they *have* been loose lately. I was eating lunch and talking to my friend Myra and suddenly they came out of place, and before I knew it I had swallowed them. I was afraid they were going to get stuck, but I could feel them gradually going down . . . you know, like an ice cube?"

I nodded.

"What will happen now?"

"Well, Mrs. Kovar, just about everything that manages to get swallowed somehow finds its way out in a few days. Even sharp or irregular objects, like straight pins and open safety pins, will go through without complications."

She gave me a brave, disbelieving smile. "Tell me the worst thing that can happen, Doctor."

I was too tired to argue, so I obliged her. "Well, your dentures could get stuck, and punch a hole in the intestine, and your stool would leak out, and you'd die."

"*What?*"

"You asked me the *worst* thing, Mrs. Kovar. It's certainly not the most likely. The most likely thing is that you'll pass them without any problems. You're not having pain or discomfort now, are you?"

"No."

"Good. Don't take any laxatives or enemas in the hope of speeding things up. If you should develop abdominal pain or cramps, come back here immediately or go to your own doctor. But they should pass safely within four to five days. If they haven't, we'll repeat the X-ray and see what progress they've made."

I started to leave.

"Doctor?"

I turned.

"How will I know whether I passed them or not?"

"Well, Mrs. Kovar, it's like this. You're going to have to check your stool every day until you find them. Use an ordinary kitchen strainer."

"Oh, Doctor. . . . No . . ."

"I'm sorry, but that's what you're going to have to do—unless you know someone who will do it for you."

She continued to stare at me helplessly.

I tried to steer her toward pleasanter thoughts. "Once you find your dentures, just clean them off and you'll be all set to eat corn-on-the-cob again."

She shook her head slowly. "Oh, I couldn't ever use them again. Not ever."

"Well, that's up to you. Right now, there's really nothing you can do except wait. Watch television, read a good book. Maybe that will help pass the time." I restrained myself from adding, "and other things."

She sighed and nodded.

Alice stuck her head around the curtain. "Dr. Nebulon is on the phone."

I left Mrs. Kovar with Alice telling her everything was going to be all right and went to talk to our cardiologist. "Dr. Nebulon, I have a sixty-three-year-old man who was brought into our emergency room in full cardiac arrest. With CPR and drugs, we got him going again. He's in a nice sinus rhythm with a blood pressure of 110 over 70. He's unconscious and not breathing, so he is currently intubated and his breathing is triggered only by the machine."

"Okay. Put him up in the unit. I have several patients to finish up with, then I'll be by to see him."

"Will do. Thanks."

When I hung up the phone, Alice was waiting. Sometimes I think Alice is always waiting.

"Dr. Sword, Mr. Gootee's wife is here. Would you talk to her? She looks like she's going to fall apart."

I told Alice to take Mrs. Gootee into the doctor's room while I finished writing on her husband's chart.

When I went in, I saw a small, tired-looking woman in her late fifties sitting on a chair that looked too big for her. "Mrs. Gootee, I'm Dr. Sword. Has anyone talked to you about your husband?"

"No. I saw one of the paramedics outside. He just said Al became ill while they were taking him to County Hospital, so they brought him here. Nothing has happened to him, has it? I mean, he's going to be all right, isn't he?"

"I'm sorry, Mrs. Gootee. Your husband did suffer a heart stoppage. We managed to get it beating again, but he's unconscious and he's not breathing on his own. The outlook isn't good."

"Oh, dear God, it's all my fault. I kept making him go to County Hospital to stop his drinking. He said his uncle died there, and he was always afraid to go there. Don't let him die. Please?"

"We're doing the best we can, Mrs. Gootee. I've called a heart specialist, Dr. Nebulon. He's coming in."

She didn't seem to hear me. "John's a good man, Doctor. It's been rough the past few years. It all started when he hurt his back. Nothing stopped the pain, so he drank to forget it. The company never did pay, not one cent. He hurt his back in the first place lifting all those heavy boxes for them. And then they fired him for drinking. He didn't used to be like this. He was a hardworking man, wouldn't take any handouts. Wish you could . . . have known him then, Doctor. Wish you could have known him then . . ." Her voice trailed off.

I got up slowly and put my hand on her shoulder. "I am sorry, Mrs. Gootee."

She was crying when I left.

I *had* to leave. I could feel tears starting up in my own eyes. I pretended to blow my nose, which I'm always doing anyway. You would think it would get easier, telling people their husband or wife or child or fiancé or mother or father has passed away, or is critically ill or injured. Instead, it seems to get harder. Maybe having watched my own father die has something to do with my feelings. Maybe it gets harder because, as time passes, I feel closer to death myself. So after I say the words "I'm sorry," I can't seem to hang around very long.

"Any man's death diminishes me, because I am involved in mankind," wrote the poet John Donne. Sometimes I think poets and doctors have a lot in common.

5

Always Look Twice

IF I HAD TO CHOOSE one area of emergency medicine that presents more, and potentially graver, problems for the EM physician than any other, I would probably have to say accidents.

Why? Did you ever hear the story of the juggler who had too many oranges? Do you remember the Sorcerer's Apprentice, trying to cope with all those buckets of water? Well, the Sorcerer's Apprentice and I had a lot in common the night my emergency room was visited by the Highland Park High School Band.

It was around 10 P.M., just after the Thursday night high-school football game had ended. The yellow school bus carrying forty-five band members and one parent chaperone started to pull out of the parking area next to the high school stadium. A gang of students whose team had just lost to Highland Park saw it, and members of the gang picked up rocks and started throwing them at the faces they believed were leering at them from behind the bus windows. The windows shattered, blood began to flow, and the terrified bus driver headed his bus toward the hospital—where, having just stitched up a bartender's lacerated finger, I was anticipating a fairly calm and uneventful evening.

As one hysterical parent and forty-five angry or sobbing or bleeding (sometimes all three) teenagers disembarked and headed toward my calm, quiet emergency room, I considered the possibility that World War III had broken out.

Whenever I am confronted with multiple accident victims, there are four problems I have to solve all at once:

I have to decide which of all those involved in the accident is the most seriously injured. In this case, practically all of the forty-five teenagers were screaming bloody murder, and I understood why. It's extremely hard for anyone who has been hurt by—or frightened in—an accident to take the time to understand that somebody else might have been hurt more. Often in situations like this there are parents or other relatives present, clamoring to have their loved one taken care of immediately. Locked into their own anxiety, they don't even hear you when you say something like, "The person over here has been more seriously injured, so I have to take care of him first." Fortunately, during the episode of the Highland Park High School Band bus, I had only one parent there in the beginning. But I knew more would soon be on their way.

I also have to decide which injuries are the most serious ones. Accident victims frequently have multiple injuries, and the most obvious injury may not be the most severe one. For example, an accident victim may have a severely cut face and also be bleeding internally. It is all too possible that while I am examining that face and wondering how fast I can move on to the girl who is screaming on the adjacent bed, I will miss the signs that would tell me the patient is bleeding internally.

When the accident victims are minors, I need parental consent to treat their injuries, or I may find myself the object of a lawsuit. To treat a minor without consent of the parents can constitute an assault. It has struck me more than once, when Alice is unable to reach a parent, how frequently today's children are left to fend for themselves. You ask the children where their parents are and they say matter-of-factly, "I don't know; I don't know when they'll be home." I think it's symbolic of the malaise of our times that most of today's kids know what's on television at any given hour of the day or night, but many of them have no idea where their parents are. Occasionally, the kids are runaways, and they don't want me—or anyone—to know it. When they say they don't know where their parents are, they neglect to add that they haven't seen them for a couple of months. Of course, if a minor is in a life-threatening emergency I'll provide whatever is necessary to sustain life. But if a minor has a simple laceration, or even a broken arm, I wait until I have parental consent. And if parental consent isn't forthcoming within a reasonable period of time, I send the child to County Hospital. It's pretty hard to sue a county hospital.

My fourth problem (which, fortunately, I didn't have to cope with that night) is the police. Police are summoned to the scene of most accidents, and they frequently accompany accident victims to the hospital, often adding confusion and fear to an already overwrought atmosphere. Some—not all, but some—will walk into the emergency room as if they owned the place: asking questions so they can finish making out their accident reports, trying to find out who was guilty of a traffic violation, or attempting to discern who was under the influence of liquor and/or drugs. Sometimes when I'm in the very process of trying to determine how seriously injured an accident victim is, the police will be pressing me to take a blood sample so they can check for blood alcohol, finish their report, and file a DWI (driving-while-intoxicated) charge.

Those are the four general varieties of problems that can accompany multiple accident victims into my emergency room.

Fortunately, in this case none of the children was critically injured. One boy who stopped a rock with his forehead was briefly unconscious (for that short period he was the only quiet one in the bunch) and we treated him first. Seven had nasty lacerations, and we managed to get parental consent over the phone to treat them. The families all had to be called to come down and pick up their children.

Alice got so harried she even stopped telling parents their sons or daughters were going to be just fine. And as the parents started arriving and milling around the emergency room until there was Standing Room Only, Shirley stopped smiling; Gloria (who is constantly on a diet) returned repeatedly to the refrigerator for a munchie to shore up her ability to cope; and Mark, who had been trying to keep a dozen or so teenage instrumentalists entertained by demonstrating various karate holds (and when that didn't work, by telling ghost stories, and when that didn't work . . .) slunk away down the corridor before I could stop him.

Even so, the Highland Park High School Band incident—with all its attendant pandemonium and confusion—wasn't as bad as what happened with Howard Rigler. I'd rather have forty-five bruised brass-band players any day than one Howard Rigler.

Moments before I met him, Howard was cruising down Warren Avenue on his big red, white, and blue Harley Davidson 750 motorcycle, when a taxicab driver made a sharp right turn and forced him off the road. Howard's cycle missed a stately tree at the side of the road, but Howard didn't.

The paramedics on duty that day were a team I call "the trophy hunters." They drove their ambulance through the streets as if they were stalking big game in Africa. Every time they wheeled a patient in on their gurney, it was as if they were presenting me with a set of horns they wanted mounted on the wall.

"Hey, Doc," one of them said as they wheeled Howard through the doors, "look at the badly fractured leg we brought you."

Already that night, things hadn't been going too well. Not a little annoyed, I asked, "Why didn't you call first?"

"Aw, hell, we didn't want to tie up the frequency for a little old broken leg," one of them said.

"He was conscious when we got to him, and he's been talking good ever since," the other added.

Right away the tone was set that nothing serious was wrong with Howard.

Gloria told the paramedics to put him in the back on bed 7—the cubicle farthest away from the critical care area. She undressed him, took his vital signs, and then left him while she put a dressing on another patient's knee. Alice came in, got all the information she needed, and had Howard sign the consent-to-treat forms for her.

As usual, I had my ears open, and nothing seemed wrong. I was busy writing on several other patients' charts, and it was a good fifteen to twenty minutes before I walked over to him and said, "Hi, Howard. How are you feeling?"

"My leg is killing me, Doc. And I can't seem to breathe right. Can't you give me a shot to knock me out?"

The second thing he said, about not being able to breathe right, should have flashed in my mind like a red beacon light. But I'd already had several complicated cases that night. I was "battle-weary," and my attention was focused a lot more on the air splint the paramedics had placed around Howard's leg than it was on what he was saying.

"Sorry, Howard. Can't give you a shot just yet. Now take it easy. I'm going to let the air out of your splint so that I can have a better look at your leg."

"It's broken all to hell, Doc."

He was right about that. I stood looking down at what had once been a tibia but now looked like a broken, oozing bamboo pole that someone had laid on top of a knee.

As I stood glumly contemplating his shattered leg, Howard suddenly grabbed my arm. "I can't breathe, Doc, I can't breathe!"

For the first time, I looked at him instead of at his leg. His breathing *was* labored. And he was starting to look "blue."

"Gloria," I yelled. "Get my stethoscope!" She brought it on the run and I listened to his lungs. The breath sounds on the right side of his chest were a lot weaker than those on the left.

"Move him down to bed number one," I ordered. "Start a critical flow sheet. Call X-ray and tell them we need a portable chest plate *stat!* Start him on oxygen at four liters per minute. And get an IV into him with Ringer's lactate."

As everybody around me moved into action, I could almost hear the voice of one of my medical school professors: "Randall, always, always check the airway, breathing, and circulation *first*."

When everything I ordered had been done, Gloria was finally able to ask, "What's happening with him?"

"His right lung isn't exchanging air," I said. "Either it's full of blood or it's collapsed. I should have looked at his leg last, not first. I know better." I shook my head.

"Well, his blood pressure's stable, so he can't have lost too much blood," she said soothingly.

I wasn't about to let myself off the hook. "I still should have checked his breathing before I checked his leg. Most people—and certainly most healthy young males—can lose a pint, even two pints of blood without losing pressure," I said. "Plus the fact that he's lying down, which tends to keep the blood pressure up. If you stood him up and the blood pooled into his legs, his pressure would become a much more sensitive indicator of blood loss."

That's why people sometimes feel faint or dizzy when they first stand up after they've been lying down for a while. The blood runs down and pools in their legs, so their blood pressure drops off.

All the time I was talking, thinking, I was watching Howard closely. Now that he was getting some oxygen, he was starting to look better to me. Not good, but better.

You can usually tell when people aren't getting enough oxygen by their behavior. They can be mildly agitated, like Howard; they can be hyperactive (in which case it's extremely dangerous to sedate them); or they can be lethargic, placid, agreeable, "good" patients.

Howard's chest X-ray revealed why he wasn't breathing too well: He had a hemothorax. The right half of his chest was filled with blood. Either the handlebars on his motorcycle or part of the tree must have hit his chest and broken several ribs, pushing sharp, needlelike edges of bone into his lungs and lacerating several arteries.

The lung is a lot like a balloon: It can be collapsed by being punctured, or compressed by blood leaking out between the rib cage and the lung. Howard's right lung had collapsed.

To treat a collapsed lung, I have to insert one end of a soft plastic tube about as thick as my little finger between the ribs and the lung. The other end of this tube leads to a vacuum pump that sucks the blood out of the lung so that the lung will re-expand to fit inside the rib cage.

I have to get the patient to hold still while I insert the tube—which isn't easy, because when I stick it in, it hurts like hell.

Howard was becoming restless and confused again, because his brain wasn't getting enough oxygen. I knew I had to work fast. I told him, "Howard, you have a chest full of blood. I have to put in a tube to drain it off. It's going to hurt, but you *must* hold still!"

I cleaned the area under his right arm and gave him a shot of Novocain to numb the area as much as I could. I made an incision half an inch long just above the sixth rib and directly under his arm in order to miss the nerve, artery, and vein that lie just under each rib. After inserting a large, curved hemostat clamp into the incision, I spread apart the fat layers and began working my way through the three layers of muscle that lie at right angles to each other between the ribs.

Then I said to Gloria, "Get those paramedics back in here to hold his arms down so he can't grab the tube after I have it in place."

Again I spoke to Howard, "Try to take a deep breath and hold it." But the lack of oxygen was getting to him. I knew he didn't understand what I was saying or doing.

Gloria came back with the paramedics. One of them held his right arm down, the other one the left.

As I pushed the last layer of muscle aside, I felt a slight give to the clamp. I was almost through. Howard screamed, and I knew I had touched the surface of the lung itself. I pushed the plastic tube through the hole I had made in his chest. Blood came pouring out from the wound onto the sheets and the floor, soaking the bottom of my pants. Even my shoes were covered with blood. It was as though a blood-filled balloon had burst—a full quart must have gushed out.

I glanced up at Gloria.

"His blood pressure is falling," she said.

"Open up his IV all the way," I told her, "and start another one in his other arm. Then have someone from the lab come over here and crossmatch him for two pints of blood."

Whenever a patient is bleeding profusely, I take ten cc's of his blood and get it typed and crossmatched for four to six pints, or units, of blood. Under normal conditions, this requires a good forty minutes. Typing the blood determines which of the major groups (types) the blood belongs to: O, A, B, or AB; and whether it's RH negative (−) or RH positive (+). These blood groups are not equally divided among the world's population. Some blood types are rare, like AB−; only 5 percent of the population has AB− blood. So if a heavy bleeder who is AB− comes in, we might have to put calls out all over the city, and even make an appeal on radio and television for that type of blood. If we're desperate and can't locate a specific blood type, we will give type O−, but this can be hazardous. Type O− is the "universal donor," which simply means that most (not all) people can be given this type of blood without having a fatal reaction.

It wasn't even known that different blood types existed until about eighty years ago, although transfusions were given long before that. The first controlled transfusions took place in 1795, when the blood of young boys was transfused into old men to try to make them live longer. Instead, a lot of them died quicker.

It wasn't until World War I that we figured out why blood transfusions produced such mixed results, saving some soldiers but killing others. Now we know that with the exception of type O−, blood types cannot be mixed without death resulting.

Crossmatching is done after a patient's specific blood type is found. A sample of the recipient's blood is mixed with a crossmatch of the donor's blood to confirm that the two bloods really will be compatible.

People used to think race determined blood type. But all of the different blood types are found among all of the different races. If you need blood, it doesn't matter whether you get it from an Indian, a black, or a Caucasian, as long as it's the right blood group.

Shirley and Mark had finished with their other patients and had come to help us with Howard.

"Here," I said to Shirley, "finish setting up the vacuum pump while I sew this suction tube to his chest."

Then I told Mark, "Get some arm restraints and tie his arms down so that he won't pull out his IVs and chest tube."

A lot of people with some degree of medical sophistication are aware that bleeding in the extremities can be controlled with external pressure alone. But with bleeding inside the chest, external pressure is impossible. After you drain off the blood, you hope the lung will re-expand and seal off the bleeding artery. This works 90 percent of the time. But in the other 10 percent, the chest has to be opened and the artery found and tied off.

Another way of controlling bleeding is by using a military

anti-shock trousers (MAST) suit, also known as a G suit. This is a vinyl bag that is wrapped around the patient just below the ribs and extends to the feet. It's very much like a large blood-pressure cuff. Air is introduced into the vinyl bag, thereby building up pressure, which in turn is controlled by a water U-tube. A MAST suit can control subdiaphragmatic bleeding by shunting blood from below the diaphragm to organs above, which are more important. Blood is, in effect, squeezed out of the lower half of the body and given to the upper half. This technique was developed by the military to use on wounded soldiers who were bleeding heavily but who had to wait one or two hours to be seen by a doctor. The MAST suit is finding more use even in cities where paramedics can reach victims within five minutes, start an IV, and arrive at the hospital within another fifteen minutes. By inflating just the legs of the MAST suit, we can auto-transfuse the patient's own blood from the legs into the trunk and head. This results in 700–1000 cc's of blood. If we then inflate the abdominal portion of the body, an additional 500 cc's or one unit of blood is squeezed into the chest and head. So the patient immediately gets two to three units of his own blood just by our inflating the suit. This is only a temporary measure to gain time until the operating team can take over. It is not a treatment.

"How's his pressure doing now?" I asked Gloria.

"It's 115 over 75, with a pulse of 110," she answered.

"How much Ringer's has gone into the IVs?"

"We have 800 cc's in the first and 400 cc's in the second."

"All right. Slow the IVs down to TKO" (to keep open; if the IV doesn't continue to drip or run at a slow pace, it will coagulate with blood). "Continue taking his pressure every fifteen minutes. If it drops below 80 mm, then we'll open the IVs again. That way, we can tell whether he's still bleeding or not."

I turned to Shirley. "How much blood has come out of the chest tube?"

"A good 600 cc's, but it's slowing down now."

"Okay. Get X-ray back in here to shoot another chest film so we can check the placement of the tube. And tell them we'll want a couple of shots of his leg while they're at it."

I left Howard with my competent staff and went out to the admitting desk.

"Alice, who's our backup thoracic surgeon on call today?"

"Just a second, I'll look."

I glanced at the clock above her desk while she thumbed through her list. Lord, I'd only been on duty a few hours. It seemed like a few years.

"Dr. Hardy," Alice said.

"Give him a call."

She nodded. As I started to walk away, I didn't get quite one full step before she said, "Uh . . . Dr. Sword? Are you terribly busy right now?"

I shrugged. "Depends on how you look at it. I still seem to have time to breathe."

"Yes, well, a mailman came in with a dog bite quite a while ago. Could you take a look at him?"

"Put him on bed three," I told her, calculating that while she was doing that I could maybe grab a quick glass of orange juice.

"He's already on bed three," she said. "I put him there an hour ago."

What was the mailman's motto? Neither sleet nor hail nor snow . . . Hell, I decided, if they could do it, so could I. I picked up his chart and walked back to see him.

"Mr. Hennessey? I'm Dr. Sword. Let's see where the dog bit you."

"Right here, Doc. Right on the back of my leg. Didn't even see the damn dog. Came right up behind me. Don't get me wrong —I love animals, Doc. I never get bitten! I think they can sense I'm a friend. I even carry dog biscuits in my pocket. But I didn't see this one, didn't have a chance to show him I was his friend. Attacked me from behind, he did."

I looked down at the wound. There were several deep punctures, and judging by the separation between them, they had been made by a good-sized dog.

"Thought he was going to take the old leg off, Doc. If he had just slowed down, I would've showed him how I wanted to be his friend."

"Well, it doesn't need stitching," I reassured him, realizing that his ego had probably received more damage than his leg. "I'll just clean it up and put a bandage on it."

If an animal bite is long and deep with jagged edges, I will clean the wound (the medical term for this is *debridement*), trim the edges, and apply a bandage. Some doctors think that bite wounds should be left open to heal from the bottom up because they are often dirty and will become infected if closed. Others believe in trimming the edges and cleaning the wound as thoroughly as possible, then sewing it up in order to get it healing faster and to minimize the size of the scar. If infection does occur after a wound is stitched, the doctor simply takes out the stitches, opens it up, and lets it heal.

Animal bites vary greatly in size and severity, depending on the size (and temperament) of the critter involved. Cat bites are similar to needle punctures, but dog bites are like slashes. Both have a high rate of infection, but the bite with the highest infection rate is a human bite. Human bites invariably get infected, so we always leave them open. If the resulting scar is too large, plastic surgery can be performed six to twelve months after the wound has healed completely. Most human bites are on the hand, but I've seen bitten ears and noses, and even breasts and penises.

"What about rabies?" Mr. Hennessey asked worriedly as I was cleaning up his wound. "Am I going to need rabies shots?"

I was able to reassure him that he probably wouldn't. If he had been bitten by a skunk, bat, or squirrel, it would have been a different story. But there hasn't been a case of rabies from a dog in the city where I practice for well over twenty years. Of course if a dog had attacked him without provocation (and unfortunately mailmen just by being mailmen provoke certain dogs), we would have put the dog under quarantine for two weeks to be certain that it *didn't* have rabies. But if it had been a wild animal and we were unable to trap and test it, we would have to go ahead with the twelve-shot rabies series.

Any mammal, even a cow, can carry rabies. The disease is caused by a virus that attacks the central nervous system (the brain and spinal cord). After the virus enters the body through a break in the skin, it will travel up the nerves and into the brain.

The farther the bite is from the brain, the longer it takes before the symptoms begin to manifest themselves. Bites to the head and neck incubate for a few weeks, while bites to the legs can take up to a year to produce symptoms. But once the virus takes hold and the victim starts to come down with the symptoms, it's too late to give the shots. Rabies is then 100 percent fatal.

I had finished bandaging Mr. Hennessey's leg and was about to wish him godspeed on his appointed rounds when Alice stuck her head around the edge of the curtain to tell me that she had Dr. Hardy on the phone.

Dr. Hardy is not one of my favorite people, and I wasn't expecting much as I picked up the phone and said, "Dr. Hardy, this is Dr. Sword at Memorial. We have a problem here, and I hope you can help us out."

"Am I on call?"

"*Am I on call?*" Jesus, I could scarcely believe he said that. I promised myself for the hundredth time to make certain no good, paying patient ever went his way.

"Yes, Dr. Hardy, you are definitely on call," I said in tones so honeyed I put Alice to shame. Then I got serious. "We have a twenty-one-year-old male who suffered a broken leg and a hemothorax in a motorcycle accident. I put in a chest tube and we've collected 800 cc's of blood out of it. His pressure dropped to 90 over 60, but we poured in lactated Ringer's and got it back up to 110 over 80. We have him typed and crossmatched for four units of blood."

"Does he have insurance?"

On hearing that question voiced before any other, letting fly with a few choice expletives would have done *me* a whole lot of good . . . but not my patient, so I stuck with the facts. "Insurance? I don't know. Let me check." I glanced at Alice. She shook her head and made a circle with her thumb and middle finger to indicate that he didn't have a job, either.

"No, no insurance," I told Dr. Hardy. "And he's unemployed."

"Well, he's stable now, isn't he?" Dr. Hardy said. "Why don't you ship him over to County?"

"Dr. Hardy, this man has a chest tube in him. His pressure has already dropped off once, he's still actively bleeding in his chest, and he has a badly fractured leg. I just don't feel we can transfer him across town at this time. I don't even think County would accept a transfer like this."

There was a long pause at the other end of the line, and then: "Well, I guess you nailed me on this one. I'll be in shortly."

I hung up the phone and shook my head. "Nailed him." The nine-to-five, don't-bother-me-on-my-lunch-hour-or-during-my-golf-game doctor. Probably by his standards, I *had* nailed him.

"Dr. Sword?" Gloria's voice summoned me back to Howard's bedside. His blood pressure was dropping off again. I told her to turn up the IVs and check with the lab to see when the blood would be ready.

Hearing some loud squalls, I glanced over my shoulder. Alice was beckoning me anxiously to the desk. "Dr. Sword, we have a two year old who caught his finger in a car door. And a Mrs. Whitmore with a migraine headache."

I could imagine how the two year old's screaming was affecting the migraine headache.

"Send the child over for X-rays," I told Alice. "And put the headache in the GYN room with the lights off."

As I scanned Mrs. Whitmore's chart, Gloria came to the desk to tell me that the lab had promised that Howard's blood would be ready in ten minutes. "When it gets here," I told her, "pump it in as fast as it will go, then call the intensive care unit and tell them Howard will be up shortly—with Dr. Hardy as the admitting physician."

I started down the corridor to see Mrs. Whitmore. Headaches are one of my least favorite maladies, because there's nothing to see. I can see a cut or a broken bone, I can see penumonia on an X-ray, I can see a heart attack on an EKG. But when patients tell me they have a headache, I can't *see* anything wrong.

Headaches can stem from a bewildering variety of causes, from benign ones, like tension, anxiety and hunger . . . to more grave ones, like meningitis, tumors, and burst blood vessels in the brain. The vast majority are not serious and will go away with aspirin and bed rest.

Mrs. Whitmore had told Alice that she had a *migraine* headache. In my opinion, migraine headaches are a great "waste-paper basket" diagnosis. People who have severe headaches automatically think they have migraine headaches. It isn't enough just to have a headache; it has to be a "migraine" headache.

The term *migraine* refers to periodic, usually one-sided throbbing headaches that first appear in childhood or early adult life and diminish with advancing years. There often is a preliminary phase, known as the *aura*, which occurs a few minutes before the headache begins. This aura can be anything from a slight disturbance in vision or speech to something as severe as semiparalysis.

Few people have true migraine headaches, but many seem to want to have their headaches labeled "migraine." And many physicians will oblige them—which is understandable, if not entirely ethical. Dr. Marcus Welby would certainly understand it: He always labels ailments. It reassures the patient, and it makes the doctor look good. After all, it sounds damned unprofessional to tell Mrs. Whitmore, "I'm not sure what's causing your headache . . ." Even if it happens to be true.

I chatted briefly with Mrs. Whitmore and gave her a physical exam to rule out any of the possible grave causes for her headache. Then I told Shirley to give her a shot for her pain. It was the easy way out for me—but my mind was still on Howard.

I went back to check on him and arrived just as the blood was going in.

"How's the pressure doing?" I asked Gloria.

"It's come up again."

"Good. Start the second pint as soon as the lab sends it down, and order two more units."

I started for my office but didn't quite make it to the door before I was stopped by a technician from X-ray. Behind him was a woman holding a small boy with a tear-stained face.

I took the X-ray and held it up to a lighted view box, studied it for a minute, then turned to the mother. She had red hair and a pleasant, freckled face. Her child clung to her as if she were the Rock of Gibraltar. After a while in this business, you begin to intuit which parents are prone to hysteria and which ones aren't, and I knew this one wasn't. I glanced at the name on the X-ray. "Mrs. Stanton?"

She nodded. "And this is Christopher."

"Well, you can relax," I said. "Christopher doesn't have a broken finger. But the nail is almost torn off, so I'll have to remove it. I'm going to numb his finger with Novocain first, so he won't feel any pain."

Removal of a fingernail or toenail is an easy procedure, and a very minor one. A fingernail will grow back in about three months, a toenail in about six.

"May I stay with him?" Christopher's mother asked me.

I nodded. The boy scarcely moved, and everything went very smoothly.

Sometimes in order to keep children still while we work on them, we end up wrapping them in sheets, or tying them to papoose boards. More than anything else, kids are just plain scared. Their pain stops once they get the initial shot of Novocain, but by then they're already in a panic and can't be calmed down.

If children are four or older, I explain exactly what I'm going to do. I tell them when they will feel pain and when they won't. Children older than seven are usually pretty good. With children between four and seven, I get mixed results. Some kick and scream regardless of what I'm doing to them; others cry at the beginning, then stop. With children three or under, I expect trouble—and usually get it.

Sometimes the parents are worse than their kids. I have seen ones who faint, or get sick, or run for the door. But this mother was a jewel. She didn't try to touch the sterile field where I was working, or keep asking me pointless questions. She just stood by her son and talked to him softly. When I was finished, I gave her an appreciative glance.

"All done, Mrs. Stanton. The nurse will put a dressing on it, and we'll see you in two days."

Dr. Hardy was waiting for me when I left Christopher's cubicle. "Howard's pressure dropped off again," I told him, "but now it's climbed back up, and he's getting his first unit of blood. The rest you know."

He nodded and went to look at Howard.

Now that he had assumed complete responsibility, I was free to give my full attention to any other problems that might arise.

Ideally, only one seriously ill or injured person will require my full attention at any one time, but often it does not work out that way. And during times when I have to divide my attention between two or three critical patients, I know it is impossible for me to do as good a job as I could if I were able to take each one separately. When I have to divide my attention, I'm always afraid I'll miss something. And so I was glad to see even good old Dr. Hardy, because if another critical patient came through those doors, I could give that person my full attention.

It wasn't long before that happened, as long, in fact, as it took me to walk into the doctor's room, sit down on the edge of the cot, and heave a deep sigh.

Then Alice stuck her head in to tell me the trophy hunters had returned. I nodded stoically and went out to meet them.

They grinned at me happily. "Hi, Doc," one said. "Got a little T.A. [traffic accident] here for you." And the other one added, "His name is John Pitt. He took out one of McDonald's golden arches with his heavy Chevy."

As they transferred Mr. Pitt from their gurney onto an empty bed, I leaned over him. "Mr. Pitt? How do you feel?"

He grimaced. "How should I feel after totaling my car?"

"Do you have any pain?"

"My left side hurts."

I checked him over carefully. One Howard Rigler in a day was enough. But Mr. Pitt was breathing fine, and he was alert. He knew what had happened and where and who he was. His pulse was 92, his blood pressure 135 over 80. He could move his extremities well, the pupils of his eyes were equal in size and constricted nicely to light, and his reflexes were normal. Because there was a possibility of heavy bleeding intra-abdominally, I ordered that some of his blood be taken (for typing and cross-matching), and some urine.

I also ordered an initial hematocrit. Hematocrit is the ratio (expressed in percentage) of red blood cells to serum, the clear portion. Normally for males it is 42 to 48 percent. For females it is 38 to 44 percent, this lower percentage being due, probably, to the blood loss during the menstrual cycle (about one-half cup every month).

Mr. Pitt's initial hematocrit was 46 percent. However, the initial hematocrit isn't an adequate indicator of any immediate blood loss that is taking place, because the ratio of red blood cells to serum takes up to a day to equilibrate. If a patient were to lose a pint of blood in five minutes his hematocrit would drop five to six percentage points, but it will take twenty-four hours to do so. It will drop 3 percent in the first eight hours; 2 percent more in the next eight hours, and an additional 1 percent during the final eight hours. Right after an accident, it's the trend we have to watch for.

While the lab work was "cooking," I sent Mr. Pitt for X-rays of his left rib cage.

"What do you think they'll find?" Shirley asked as he was being wheeled away.

"I suspect he might have some broken ribs over his kidney on the left side," I said.

"If there's been any kidney damage, blood will show up in his urine, won't it?" she asked.

"Yes," I said, "but the amount of blood in the urine doesn't necessarily correlate with the extent of the damage."

"What do you mean?"

"Well, for example, a football player who suffers a bruised kidney in a game will show a few red cells in his urine. This isn't serious, and they'll be gone in a day or two. But a person whose kidney has been broken in half from a severe blow might also show only a few red blood cells in the urine.

"The opposite can be true, too. Blood might be literally pouring from the penis, and the accident victim may have only a small tear in the kidney or bladder—which will repair itself if left alone. Then again, the bladder could be ruptured totally. So the amount of blood in the urine doesn't necessarily reflect the seriousness of the injury."

As Shirley opened her mouth to ask me another question, Gloria poked her head out from one of the curtained areas and motioned me over urgently. A little girl I judged to be about ten was lying on the bed. A woman I assumed was her mother grabbed my sleeve. "Oh, Doctor, help my little girl!" Clearly, I wasn't going to be lucky enough to get two nonhysterical parents in a row.

"What happened?" I asked Gloria.

"I gather Lisa was walking atop a picket fence—balancing, you know, on the cross beam—when a dog frightened her. She fell, and caught the fence between her legs."

I gently disengaged the mother's hand from my sleeve. "Maybe you'd better step outside while I examine your daughter."

She looked at me as if I'd asked her to go to Siberia.

"All right. But please stand over there against the wall."

Clearly reluctant, she did as I asked. Then I looked down at the girl. "Lisa, I'm Dr. Sword. I need to see the place where you're hurt."

Lisa didn't say a word, just kept her eyes on the ceiling and let me look. Between her legs, just to the left of the vagina, was an ugly round black-and-blue mark. There was a trickle of blood from the vagina.

The mother came up behind me and started moaning, "She's lost her virginity, hasn't she, Doctor? I knew it, I just knew it!"

I'd known, of course, that that mother wouldn't stay put against the wall. I had to restrain myself from snapping the woman's head off. I managed to mutter, "Of course not."

The hymen, a thin membrane of skin at the entrance to the vagina, is often broken by bicycling, horseback riding, or even doing acrobatic splits. But a broken hymen does not constitute a loss of virginity. I began to talk softly to the girl. "Lisa, I want to check your urine and get some X-rays. If these are okay, then we'll put you to bed for a few days with an ice pack. All right?"

With her solemn eyes still resolutely fastened on the ceiling, she nodded.

When I had finished with Lisa, Mr. Pitt's urine-test results and X-rays were ready for me to read. The urinalysis showed a few red cells, the X-rays revealed two fractured ribs, numbers 11 and 12, on the left side—near where the left kidney is located.

I went to talk to him. "Mr. Pitt, I'm worried about your left kidney. I'd like you to sign a consent form to allow us to do an intravenous pyelogram."

"I already signed a consent form when I came in."

"That was a consent-to-treat form," I explained. "It only authorizes us to do normal things like lab work and X-rays. In order to perform any special procedure, I need you to sign a specific form for it."

"Yeah, well, what is this intra . . . intra . . ."

"IVP is what we call it for short," I said. "We inject a small amount of dye into a vein in your arm. As the dye circulates through your body, it is picked up and concentrated by the kidneys. If a kidney is damaged, we're able to see it on the X-ray. We'll take X-rays after five, ten, fifteen, and thirty minutes, and even one hour, if necessary; we'll keep taking them until the dye shows up."

"Okay," he said. "Just so I know what I'm getting into."

As he was being wheeled out the door to X-ray, a young man came limping in. Shirley conversed with him softly for a few minutes, then came over to me.

"He's a football player," she said. "He twisted his ankle, and his coach wants him to have X-rays."

"Send him the hell over to X-ray, then," I snapped, and stalked away.

Shirley knew from past experience that my anger wasn't directed at her. This is one of my pet peeves: coaches ordering X-rays. Coaches should let doctors decide whether or not their players need X-rays. Since I'm concerned about problems with radiation, I don't like to order X-rays unless I have a good reason. When coaches tell their players to come in and get an X-ray, I feel almost forced to give them one, whether I think it's necessary or not.

My temper was nearing the ragged edge anyway. Shirley had been watching me, and she knew it. She dispatched the young man to X-ray, brought me a cup of coffee, and ordered me—with a stern scowl—to sit down and drink it. Which I did, grateful (as I often am) for the understanding of my colleagues.

When the young athlete's X-rays came back, there was no fracture or dislocation, just the soft-tissue swelling indicating a sprain. Actually, a sprained ankle can be almost as much of a problem to the person who has it as a broken one. I told the football player to elevate his ankle about six to eight inches above his heart and keep ice on it for two days, then to apply heat and start putting weight on it. Sprains usually take one to two weeks before they're much improved. I told him if it didn't start to feel better in five days, he should have it rechecked by an orthopedic surgeon.

"Will I have to have a cast if it doesn't get better?" he asked worriedly. "We've got a big game coming up."

"Depends on which doctor you go to," I answered. "Some orthopedic surgeons believe all severely sprained ankles should have a cast. Others feel that an elastic bandage is all that's necessary. And some will drain the ankle with a large needle on the second day, and shoot in Novocain and cortisone to facilitate walking."

"Yeah, well, can you give me the name of one of the ones who doesn't believe in casts?" he asked me.

Before I could answer, Shirley came to tell me John Pitt's X-rays were back. I left her to finish up with the football player and went to study the X-rays.

It is often extremely difficult to correctly diagnose trauma to the abdomen. There are so many possible organs to consider when looking for the source of pain: the liver, the spleen, the kidneys, the pancreas, the bladder—and thirty-three feet of small and large intestine.

Any sharp missile or instrument can cause a penetrating wound. Injuries to the small intestine are usually the result of penetrating wounds, like stab or bullet wounds. When the small bowel has been punctured, air can escape, rise, and lodge underneath the diaphragm, the thin muscle that separates the thoracic (chest) cavity from the abdominal cavity. This free air will show up on an X-ray.

Penetrating injuries have to be opened surgically and explored. Small penetrating wounds to the small intestine are usually simply closed by surgery, after which a suction tube can be placed in the patient's stomach, and the patient will be fed intravenously so the stomach and bowel can rest. Larger, more severe wounds may necessitate a resection. A resection can be compared to taking a leaky hose, cutting out the part that is leaking, and connecting the cut ends back together again.

Penetrating wounds of the colon (large intestine) are less frequent but more serious than those of the small intestine, because of the bacteria present in the large intestine. There's very little—if any—bacteria in the stomach or the small bowel; but the large intestine is loaded, because this is where the feces are formed and stored. It isn't necessary to localize the point of injury to the colon prior to surgery, since it's easy to see at the time of operation.

Colon injuries are managed with broad-spectrum antibiotics, with fluid and salt replacement by IVs, and with resection of the devitalized part. If the injury is in the right side of the colon, then the devitalized area is taken out and the cut ends are sutured back together immediately. If the injury is on the transverse (crossover) or the left side of the colon, where most of the contamination resides, there is more of a problem. A primary repair and closure is usually not done. Instead, the large intestine is taken out through the abdominal wall and sewn in place, but the wall is left open. A "colostomy" has been done, and the patient has a second anus coming out of the abdominal wall. It will be closed several weeks later.

Nonpenetrating wounds to the abdomen occur by forceful contact with blunt objects—for example, when a person is thrown against a steering wheel or is punched in the belly, or simply bumps into a piece of furniture. Since the damage and bleeding are on the inside, an observation period of several days may be necessary to permit accurate assessment of the situation.

Evidence of intra-abdominal injury may not become apparent for many hours or even days after the injury. A small leakage of intestinal contents may take time to cause symptoms. Blood vessels of the bowel may become blocked, causing the bowel to become necrotic (dead), and then leakage will occur days later. The patient may arrive in the emergency room with symptoms similar to a ruptured appendix with peritonitis (inflammation of the membrane that lines the abdominal cavity).

Getting a good history from the patient is vitally important in helping make a correct diagnosis. Unfortunately, this isn't always possible since the patient may be in shock, unconscious, or incoherent due to drugs or alcohol.

Abrasions and black-and-blue marks can be useful clues to the nature of the trauma. So can pain, with localized tenderness;

the absence of bowel sounds; nausea; vomiting; or swelling of the abdominal cavity.

Fracture of the lower ribs can point to possible abdominal injuries. A rib itself, once it's broken, is like a dry stick; it can puncture a kidney or one of the other organs in the abdomen, which was what had happened in Mr. Pitt's case. The dye showed a picture of a normal right kidney—three inches long, two inches wide, and one inch thick. But there was definite irregularity around the left kidney, where the dye had leaked out. As I suspected, it had been punctured by one of his broken ribs. Only an operation would reveal how much damage had been done and whether or not the damaged kidney should be removed.

I told Alice to call Dr. Coleman, a hospital urologist.

While I waited for her to get him on the line, I thought about a patient from the night before, Mr. Marshall. He was a middle-aged, heavyset man who had stopped off at his favorite tavern for a few drinks after work, and left for home without urinating. On his way home, he ran his car into a lamp pole. Upon arriving at the emergency room, he complained of lower abdominal pain. His X-rays were negative for fractures, and his blood pressure was good. But when he urinated, it was almost pure blood. The IVP showed normal kidneys and ureters (the tubes that carry urine from the kidneys to the bladder), but his bladder didn't show up too well on the X-ray.

The normal bladder is a roundish, thin, muscular sphere that is able to store up to a pint of urine (though the storage capacity greatly increases under certain conditions). Like a balloon, the walls of the bladder thin out when the bladder is full. A full balloon is easier to burst than one that is half full, and so is a full bladder. Three out of four burst bladders are associated with trauma and a fractured pelvis. However, only 15 percent of fractured pelvises have burst bladders. The moral of this story is to empty your bladder before you drive.

Interestingly enough, the female reproductive organs are rarely injured in accidents, since they are set in deep and protected by the bony pelvis, which is shaped like a shallow bowl. During the first three or four months of life, the fetus is protected by this bowl. As the fetus grows in size and emerges from the pelvic bowl, it is protected by the liquid cushion of its own sterile urine. Few accidents result in the death of a fetus without also killing the mother.

When Alice had Dr. Coleman on the line, I told him what was happening with John Pitt and got his permission to admit him to Urology.

After I hung up the phone, Alice gave me one of her maternal everything-is-going-to-be-just-fine looks. I knew what that meant. "The trophy hunters again?" I asked.

She nodded. "They're bringing in another accident victim."

I shrugged philosophically and tossed my favorite line from "Gunga Din" at her: "Better days are comin', Gunga Din."

She surprised me by chortling merrily.

Four minutes later, the trophy hunters were wheeling their latest catch through the swinging doors.

"Hello again, Doc. Keeping you busy?" said one.

I nodded, about to toss another of my favorite lines from "Gunga Din" at them; but the second paramedic beat me to the punch, saying, "I tell you, Doc, they are just cracking up to get in here and see you."

For the life of me, I couldn't think of a snappy comeback. So I focused my attention on my new patient, Phillip Liston. Like Mr. Marshall, he had collided with a lamp pole. Even though he had no obvious injuries, he seemed more ill than his vital signs indicated, and I began to get a bad feeling about him. After a few Howard Riglers, you develop a sixth sense about these things.

"Mr. Liston," I said, "I understand your car jumped a curb and hit a pole. Is that right?"

"I don't exactly remember. I was going to work; then there was a loud noise; and suddenly all these people were around me."

"Where are you now?"

"In some hospital, I guess."

"That's right. This is Memorial Hospital. Do you have any pain?"

"Only on my right side."

I examined him and found some minor tenderness under his right rib cage. I still felt uneasy about him. Just to satisfy myself, I had the nurses start an IV and get a sample of urine. I had the lab come over to draw blood for typing and crossmatching, and then I sent him over for abdominal and right-rib X-rays.

"What are you worried about?" Gloria asked. "A ruptured spleen?"

I shook my head. "Liver," I said.

The spleen is the abdominal organ most frequently injured by blunt trauma and is often associated with rib fractures on the left side. In fact, delayed rupture of the spleen may occur even two weeks after the accident, although most "delayed ruptures" are really delays in diagnosis.

Injuries to the liver, like those to the spleen, are mostly associated with blunt trauma to the abdomen and the lower chest, usually on the right side, where Mr. Liston's tenderness was.

"How do we find out for sure?" Gloria asked.

I wasn't sure how to answer her. If I were positive he had a ruptured liver, I would call a surgeon to come open up his belly and repair it. But I wasn't positive; I just had this uneasy feeling.

If a patient is bleeding internally, he or she will often become "shocky"—develop a low blood pressure because of the loss of blood. If we can't find any obviously discernible bleeding area, then we have to figure he could be bleeding from the chest, which would show up on an X-ray. If the chest isn't involved, the only other conceivable place is the abdomen. To establish whether or not abdominal bleeding is occurring, we do a paracentesis, or tapping of the abdominal cavity.

When Mr. Liston's X-rays came back, they didn't show any masses or fractured ribs. But my uneasy feeling still wouldn't go away. I went to look him over again.

"How are you doing, Mr. Liston? Still tender under the right ribs?"

He nodded. "My right shoulder hurts, too, but I seem to be able to move it okay."

Pushing down lightly on his abdomen just under the right rib cage elicited a much more significant pain response than I had gotten before.

I knew his shoulder pain could be stemming from the fact that he had calmed down and so was discovering aches and pains all over. Or it could stem from something more serious: It was possible that blood under his right diaphragm was referring pain to his right shoulder. But I didn't want to waste any more time before I found out.

"Mr. Liston," I said, "I need to find out whether you are bleeding inside your abdominal cavity. I'd like your permission to do a paracentesis. We'll insert a needle into your abdominal wall about an inch below your belly button. If any blood comes out, then we'll need to do an exploratory operation. If there is no blood, then a thin flexible-plastic tube will be inserted through the needle, and we'll put a quart of salt solution into your abdomen with it. We'll leave it there for five to ten minutes, and then siphon it off. The fluid will be examined for blood—and for bacteria from feces, which would indicate a ruptured intestine. If this test is negative, it pretty much rules out the possibility that you have serious intra-abdominal bleeding or injury. But if the test is positive, then an operation is indicated. Do you have any questions?"

He didn't feel well enough to have any questions. "No. . . . Just do what's best, Doc."

The test turned out positive, and the surgeon called to come in and open him up found a four-inch laceration in his liver. This was loosely sutured with a substance having the consistency of gelatin, since the liver doesn't hold sutures well. Mr. Liston went home nine days later.

Me, I went home as soon as the surgeon arrived to take over the care of Mr. Liston. My shift was over, and I figured I'd had enough trophies for one night.

6

Tell Me Where It Hurts

A FRAZZLED PHYSICIAN who had just come from treating a nurse once told me that nurses make terrible patients. After my encounter with Mary McGuire, I understood what he meant.

When Alice handed me the chart that Friday night, she informed me that my next patient was a surgical nurse. It's been my observation that surgeons and surgical nurses tend to have tunnel vision: they don't see medicine as a holistic concept, but concentrate exclusively on surgery. Consequently, a lot of surgeons and surgical nurses have fairly rigid personalities. So I wasn't surprised, when I entered the cubicle where Mary McGuire was waiting, to see an expression on her face reminiscent of the expressions carved on the faces on Mt. Rushmore. Nevertheless, I greeted her with my usual determined cheerfulness. "Hi, I'm Dr. Sword. What can I do for you?"

"I want some X-rays of my ribs," she snapped. Just like that; as if I were a butcher and she was ordering a roast.

I smiled, probably somewhat woodenly. "Really. Why?"

"Because I want to know," she said in that precise way certain adults have when they wish to imply that the people they are talking to are imbeciles, "if my ribs are broken."

Taking a deep breath, I asked, "And why do you think your ribs might be broken?"

"Because they hurt," she snapped.

Clearly, she was losing patience with me. But not as fast as I was losing patience with her. "Why do they hurt?" I snapped right back.

"Because I fell down."

"How? Where? When?"

She cast her eyes upward at the ceiling in a Dear-God-help-me-through-this look and said with heavy patience, "When I got up today, I fell against a sharp corner of my dresser. I didn't lose consciousness, and I don't need any blood tests. All I need is an X-ray of my ribs."

"Tell me where you hurt," I said.

"Under where my ribs are," she said sarcastically.

I didn't say a word. I just stared at her. My son Tod hates it when I do that, and it usually makes him back down.

My staring had some effect on Mary McGuire, too. Not a lot, but some. "Look," she said, "how old are you? Still in your thirties, right? I imagine I've been working in a hospital about six times as long as you have. If there's anything wrong with me, I know enough to know that it has to do with my ribs. You can understand that, can't you?"

I nodded. "Sure, Mary, I can understand that. Now if you'll lie down and tell me exactly where you hurt, I'll examine you. I want you to lie down, put your arms at your sides, bend your knees slightly, and take a deep breath."

If looks could kill, I'd have been long gone. But Mary knew hospital etiquette, and she knew when she was licked. This was my emergency room; I was the doctor in charge. She had tried to browbeat me and had failed.

I wasn't doing what I was doing because I wanted to engage her in a power play, but because I wanted to be damn sure I diagnosed correctly whatever was wrong with her. She said she had fallen. Well, what made her fall? Dizziness? Nausea? And was her fall actually responsible for her pain? The lower part of the heart rests on top of the stomach, separated from it only by the diaphragm. So for whatever reason people may think they're having upper abdominal pain, there are myriad possible explanations. Generally, we divide the abdomen into "surgical" versus "nonsurgical" conditions, but it may not always be obvious at the outset which is which.

Even a surgical nurse with a rigid personality should know that abdominal pain is one of the most mysterious problems that confront physicians. When I'm looking for the cause of an abdominal pain, it isn't enough to emulate Dr. Kildare; I have to *be* Dr. Kildare, Sherlock Holmes, and Dr. Watson all rolled up into one. And certainly a surgical nurse should know that with abdominal pain, perhaps more than with any other symptom, the history —meaning the who, what, where, when, and how—of the pain is of vital importance.

The age of the patient is a factor, because many conditions are pretty much confined to a particular age group. For example, appendicitis is most common in adolescents and young adults; only rarely does it occur in infants—in whom a much more frequent cause of severe abdominal pain is acute intussusception, which occurs when a portion of the small bowel infolds into an adjacent portion. The most common cause of intestinal obstruction in adults over forty is blockage by a cancerous stricture, and this condition is seldom seen in anyone younger than thirty. Acute pancreatitis is seldom seen in anyone under middle age; a perforated gastric ulcer is rare in anyone under fifteen. Troublesome conditions of the gallbladder, or a twisted ovarian cyst, may occur in childhood but are much more common in adults.

I judged Mary to be in her early fifties. I could rule out the probability of some things, and not others. Maybe her pain *was* being caused by broken ribs, but it was my responsibility to determine that, not hers.

Onset, or the way a pain begins, is also important in figuring out what's causing the pain. If I have a patient who states he has been awakened out of a sound sleep by a pain in his abdomen, I'm immediately alerted for trouble, because no ordinary pain begins like that. Acute appendicitis or perforation of a gastric ulcer will wake people up, as will strangulation of the gut (when it twists around itself), or an ovarian cyst. A ruptured ectopic pregnancy can be acute in onset, too. If a patient faints or falls down or collapses at the onset of the symptoms, perforation of a gastric or duodenal ulcer, acute pancreatitis, or a dissecting abdominal aneurysm (here, the pain is primarily in the back) can be considered likely possibilities. If the pain is slow in building up and vomiting is ultimately involved, an intestinal obstruction has to be considered.

And how long a pain lasts is important. It's not unusual for an appendix to perforate within the first twenty-four hours after the onset of symptoms. Therefore, if a patient describes a pain that indicates the appendix is involved and I know when that pain started, I can estimate the most probable pathological changes that have occurred if it is appendicitis, and investigate accordingly. An acute gallbladder attack doesn't usually persist for longer than two days before complications set in. Cancer of the intestinal tract, on the other hand, may be experienced as dull pain for weeks or even months before it is identified.

The location of the pain is important. Certain organs provide a reasonably circumscribed area of pain. The stomach and duodenum, for example, are quite reliable. The pain from these organs localizes between the rib cages and umbilicus in an area called the epigastrium. The pain of pancreatitis is located in the upper abdomen. Appendicitis classically causes pain in the right lower quadrant of the abdomen. Ovarian and fallopian-tube pain is in the right or left area just above the pubic bone. Gallbladder spasms show up in the right upper quadrant. Other organs, such as the small or large intestines, have poor localization; people tend to point vaguely to areas somewhere around their umbilicus.

The radiation, or reference, of pain is often helpful in making a diagnosis. Gallbladder or biliary-tract pain begins in the right upper quadrant and radiates around the right side to just beneath the shoulder blade. The pain of the pancreas radiates through to the midline of the back. Appendix pain generally starts just below the rib cage and migrates to the right lower quadrant. Kidney pain starts in the back but frequently drops down to the genital area. In certain conditions of the upper abdomen or lower chest regions, pain may be referred to the top of the shoulder or the side of the neck. This happens when blood from a ruptured spleen or acid from a perforated stomach ulcer irritates the underside of the diaphragm.

When I told Mary to bend her knees slightly, which relaxes the stomach muscles, and take a deep breath, she said, "I can't. I can't even straighten my right leg out anymore—it hurts too much. And I can't take a deep breath, because that hurts too much, too."

I began to feel pretty strongly that more than broken ribs were involved, which is why it is so important for me to ask questions and examine the patient. I have to visualize in my own head all the possibilities that match the symptoms, and listen to, look at, and touch the patient. Often it is touching that allows a genuine communicative bond to develop between the doctor and the patient, and all the extras—the lab work, X-rays, special equipment, special tests—can't replace touch.

When I examined Mary, it was evident that she had taken a pretty substantial fall. Tenderness, swelling, and bluish discoloration were already evident over her right upper side. The discoloration was caused by small blood vessels under the skin that had broken and leaked out blood.

After examining her, I did order the X-rays that she wanted—but because *I* felt they were necessary, not because she did. When I left her, she was telling the X-ray technician exactly how and where to position his X-ray machine.

Alice met me outside Mary's cubicle to inform me that while I had been arguing with Mary, an old woman—vomiting and complaining of abdominal pain—had been brought in by her family, and was waiting to see me on bed 4. I scanned her chart as I walked down the corridor. Her name was Zela Zusman, and she had been born in 1899.

Mrs. Zusman was a tiny lady with silver hair and dimples buried in her wrinkles. I suspected she was the kind of woman who didn't complain unless she had something to complain about, and then only when she was certain that whatever it was wasn't going to go away. I looked carefully at the way she was lying, because the position a patient assumes in order to obtain relief from pain can often be helpful in making a diagnosis. Victims of pancreatitis frequently lie on their side with knees and hips flexed, which relaxes the muscles that are irritated and in spasm. Patients with appendicitis often flex just the right leg and thigh in order to relax the muscles on the right. Patients with a widespread peritonitis lie very quietly and refrain from any type of movement at all. Patients with a kidney stone roll about restlessly and are uncomfortable in any position. But there are also stoic patients, who don't want to give away anything at all about where it hurts or trouble you with the fact that they're in pain. I was afraid Mrs. Zusman might be one of those.

"Mrs. Zusman?" I said. "I'm Dr. Sword. How long have you been sick?"

She half sat up as if she wanted to peek around the curtain.

I glanced over my shoulder, then back at her. "What is it?"

"Is my daughter-in-law out there?" she whispered. "Can she hear me?"

"Your daughter-in-law is in the waiting room," I said. "Nobody can hear you."

She lay back down again, relaxing, and said in a normal tone, "I've been sick about a week and a half. When it started, I thought it was my daughter-in-law's cooking. She always tries out new dishes on me before she gives them to my son. But I decided even my daughter-in-law's cooking wouldn't make me this sick."

"What kind of pain are you experiencing?"

Understanding the character of the pain is often helpful in diagnosing what's causing it. Acute abdominal pain is either constant or crampy (intermittent). Constant pain may wax and wane somewhat, but it isn't cyclic and doesn't appear in successive waves as abdominal cramps do. Constant pain is usually caused by an inflammation such as appendicitis, or by a gallbladder attack, or by cancer involving an organ. Crampy or colicky pain is usually caused by an intestinal obstruction or a kidney stone.

"I have these terrible cramps that come and go," she said. "And look at me, doctor. I'm swelling up like the Goodyear blimp."

Abdominal distention, or swelling, is best assessed by measuring the abdominal girth at the umbilicus, and by viewing the contour of the abdomen in a line between the pubic bone and the place where the bottom of the ribs come together (called the xiphoid process). In patients without swelling, the abdominal border will usually lie below the xiphoid–pubic line. Even in patients who are fat, this holds true. When the abdomen is distended, however, the line curves outward. Mrs. Zusman's abdomen was definitely distended.

Percussion (tapping on the abdomen) helps decide whether the swelling is due to gas or fluid. If there is gas, you get a tympanitic (sharp) note; if there is fluid, you get a dull note. If the fluid is present in the abdominal cavity rather than localized within the stomach or part of the intestines, you get a "shifting" dullness. The presence of fluid gives a dull note on the sides of the abdomen, while on the front it gives a tympanitic note. Turning the patient on his side changes the location of the tympanitic note to the side that is up, while the front part of the abdomen then gives a dull note. Patients with distention due to a colon (large intestine) obstruction are less likely to vomit than patients with an intestinal obstruction higher up in the small bowel, which is closer to the stomach.

"When was the last time you vomited?" I asked Mrs. Zusman.

"A couple of hours ago," she replied.

Vomiting is always an important symptom. The stimulus that causes it may originate in the brain, the inner ear, the gastrointestinal tract, or the diaphragm. Vomiting related to the intake of solid foods or beverages is likely to be a gastrointestinal problem and is usually preceded by nausea. Vomiting unaccompanied by nausea is more likely to be due to a problem in the brain. When patients with head injuries (especially children) vomit, the reason must be investigated, because the vomiting may be an indication of increasing intracranial pressure. The time of eating as related to the time of vomiting is also important. Vomiting immediately after eating suggests an esophageal problem, while vomiting shortly after eating suggests a stomach or duodenal area abnormality and vomiting between meals is more likely to be due to an intestinal obstruction. With young children, meningitis or poisoning must also be considered as possible causes.

Frequent early vomiting is present in patients with an irritation or inflammation of the pancreas, or with a perforation of the stomach or duodenum by an ulcer. It is extremely unusual for patients with acute pancreatitis *not* to vomit; in contrast, vomiting is seldom seen in acute inflammation of the gallbladder.

The character of the vomited material is of little help in making a diagnosis unless (as in the case of a low obstruction) vomiting continues until the large-bowel contents come up into the mouth. In an empty stomach, vomiting begins with yellow-colored vomitus; then as it persists bile is refluxed up into the stomach, giving the vomitus a greenish color. If vomiting persists for a long time, the odor changes from sour to foul. Eventually you get fecallike material that has backed all the way up from the large intestine.

"Where is your pain now?" I asked Mrs. Zusman.

"Mostly here." She pointed to her mid-abdomen and lower right side, circling the area with her finger.

"Does the pain go anywhere?" I asked her. "Does it seem to travel to some other place?"

"No," she replied, "it stays right there. But sometimes it gets worse."

I watched her face intently as she spoke. A patient's facial expression will occasionally furnish some clue as to the severity of the pain she is enduring. Pale or bluish skin, or a sudden grimace of pain, usually indicates that some grave abdominal catastrophe has occurred. But appearances are often deceptive, and it is only after seeing hundreds of people in pain that you begin to trust your intuition. I sensed Mrs. Zusman was experiencing a fair degree of pain.

I asked her to remain quiet while I examined her. Examination of the abdomen is probably one of the most difficult procedures to describe. It is important, when first examining a patient, to touch the area farthest removed from the point of maximum pain. Rigidity of the abdominal muscles (called "guarding") indicates spasms secondary to a nearby inflammatory process. Rebound tenderness, elicited by gently pushing down on the abdomen and then suddenly letting go, occurs in the area of maximum tenderness (and inflammation) no matter where the abdomen is pushed. The proper way to examine the abdomen is learned only by feeling literally hundreds and hundreds of abdomens.

But before I feel, I listen. I listen to the frequency and pitch of the bowel sounds. The normal frequency of the bowel in a fasting state is ten to twelve sounds of peristalsis per minute. With a localized inflammation, such as appendicitis, the intestinal sounds become less frequent. In a diffuse inflammation such as peritonitis, the bowel is more active; hence, more sounds. The "pitch" of the peristaltic sounds (sounds of the wormlike movement by which the digestive tract moves its contents) depends on the tension of the intestinal wall. Just as the pitch of a snare drum is raised by increasing the tension of the drum head, so the pitch of the bowel sounds is raised by increasing the intraluminal tension. If a bowel is paralyzed, a large amount of air and water will accumulate and cause swelling, thereby raising the pitch of the peristalsis.

A rectal examination is also necessary when trying to solve the mystery of abdominal problems. The lower third of the abdomen is hidden by the pelvic bone and can be examined only through the rectum. I once found a toothpick in the rectum of a man complaining of abdominal pain. He said he had swallowed it!

Prior to examining Mrs. Zusman, I knew only that she was suffering from a colicky midabdominal pain, nausea, and vomiting. These could be due to appendicitis, gallbladder disease, kidney stones, a twisted ovarian cyst, or a small or large bowel obstruction. After examining her, I tended to think she had a bowel obstruction. Her bowel sounds were frequent and loud; in fact, they sounded like water dropping on a tight snare drum. Her rectal examination was normal, but she appeared to be dehydrated, in a fair amount of pain, and her abdomen was visibly distended. She also had a slightly elevated temperature, which didn't surprise me. Patients with acute abdominal disease, such as acute appendicitis, an intestinal obstruction, or a ruptured ectopic pregnancy, will record a temperature of 100 degrees orally, or 101 degrees rectally. Temperatures a degree or two higher than that usually indicate a lung or urinary-tract infection rather than the involvement of an intra-abdominal process, and temperatures over 104 mean an abscess or a generalized systemic infection involving the lung, urinary tract, or nervous system. While preschool children can spike temperatures of 104 or 105 degrees at the drop of a hat because their temperature-regulating mechanism hasn't fully matured, if an adult's temperature spikes suddenly upward, it can mean the bowel has ruptured and gangrene is present.

But I wasn't as sure of Mrs. Zusman's diagnosis as I would have liked, and so I ordered some laboratory tests. Lab tests aren't often terribly helpful in diagnosing abdominal pain, but usually I will order certain ones in order to confirm or disprove my own thinking about what might be wrong, satisfy the patient and the patient's family that everything that could possibly be done is being done, and complete the record in order to "cover my ass." I'll ask for a urine test, for example, to determine whether there is sugar or any sign of infection present in the urine. And since I have learned the hard way that all women over age twelve and under age fifty are to be considered pregnant unless proven otherwise, I order a pregnancy test for that age group.

I remember once when a school nurse brought in a fourteen-year-old girl. The girl, who had been vomiting off and on for weeks, insisted nothing was wrong, but the nurse brought her in anyway. We were busy that morning, so I ordered some lab work and abdominal X-rays while I looked after the other patients. When I finally had a chance to see the films, there big as life was a twenty-six-week-old fetus. Experiences like that one have taught me always to ask women about the regularity or irregularity of their menstrual cycle and about the presence (or absence) of a vaginal discharge.

My standard order for lab tests also includes a blood test to see whether the white blood count is elevated. If it is, this will confirm that the body is experiencing stress due to an infection or an obstruction.

Even more helpful than the initial results of lab tests are the results of serial tests, which are repeated after six, twelve, or twenty-four hours. These determine whether any changes from the initial readings have gone up or down. If I'm not fairly certain of a diagnosis, I will often have a patient go home and return six to twelve hours later for a repeat of a lab test.

Mrs. Zusman's lab tests revealed no blood in her stool or vomitus. However, her white count was elevated, and I decided to order X-rays.

X-rays can be valuable diagnostically. A chest X-ray can rule out pulmonary disease or reveal air underneath the diaphragm (suggesting a perforation somewhere in the intestinal tract).

Abdominal X-rays can reveal abnormal soft-tissue densities, such as stones. Kidney stones, for example, can be seen 90 percent of the time on X-rays because they contain enough calcium to be visible.

I wanted a set of abdominal X-rays on Mrs. Zusman, but I wanted to talk to her family before I ordered them.

As I walked back up the corridor on my way to the waiting room, Alice flagged me down with Mary McGuire's X-rays. I wasn't too surprised at what I saw. When I went to tell Mary about them, she was lying quietly, her face pale and stressed with the look doubt and pain produce.

"Mary," I said, "your X-rays reveal four broken ribs on the right side." I gave her a minute to say, "I told you so," but she didn't, so I went on. "This could mean big trouble. I'm sure you've felt the ends of broken bones. You know how sharp they can be. The jagged end of a broken rib can puncture a lung as easily and as swiftly as a knife can. Your intestines could also be perforated. Your liver lies right under the lower two broken ribs, and your right kidney isn't exempt, either."

"I can't stay in the hospital," she countered firmly. "I have to go to work tomorrow. Now you just put some kind of splint or binder around my ribs, give me some pain pills, and send me on my way. That's all I came here for."

"I appreciate the fact that you want to go to work, Mary, but I wouldn't be doing *my* job if I let you walk out of here right now. Putting a binder on your ribs might reduce your pain, but at the same time, your breathing would become shallow. And as you know, when your breathing is shallow, the lungs remain partially collapsed—which underneath fractured ribs could bring on pneumonia. And frankly, I'm just damned suspicious that one of your broken ribs may have lacerated your liver. We need to start an IV, we need to type and crossmatch you for some blood, get a hematocrit and urine and maybe a liver scan. And you need to tell me your doctor's name so I can give him a call."

She pressed her lips tightly together, and I thought for a minute she wasn't going to tell me. But finally she relented.

"Dr. Kramer."

"He's a general practitioner?"

She nodded.

"You're going to need a surgical consultation, too. Do you have a general surgeon you've gone to or would like me to call?"

She gave me a wry look. "When I'm not working, Dr. Sword, I stay away from doctors as much as I can. Especially surgeons."

"I can understand that," I said, absolutely deadpan. "So I tell you what. I'll talk to Dr. Kramer and see if he has anyone he would like to recommend. If not, I'll call one of the surgeons on staff here. You just lie still, and I'll send one of the nurses in to start your IV."

"Apparently," she said, "I'm going to have a busman's holiday."

"I never met a nurse yet who couldn't use some rest," I replied. "Relax and enjoy it."

When I left Mary, I went to bring Mrs. Zusman's son and daughter-in-law back to her bedside. I like to talk to all the members of a family at one time, and inform them as much as is practical about what is being done and why.

As we all gathered together, before I had a chance to begin, the daughter-in-law said with a guilty look on her face, "It wasn't something she ate, was it?"

I shook my head. "I wish it were that simple."

"What do you mean?" the son asked.

"After talking to your mother and examining her, I believe her problem is a bowel obstruction. The most definitive test for bowel obstruction is a series of X-rays of the abdomen. We'll take one picture of your mother lying down and one sitting up. The first picture is to see if the loops of her intestine are dilated or not. The second is to see whether the loops have a fluid level like a glass half full of water. Gas is normally visible in the colon and stomach but not the small bowel. If there is an intestinal obstruction, gas collects along with retained fluid. So the gas–fluid levels in the bowel can confirm the diagnosis."

"What would cause such an obstruction?" the daughter-in-law asked worriedly.

"It could be any one of a number of things," I said. "A twisted loop of intestine, a cancerous growth, adhesions, a gallstone. She may have to undergo surgery before we find out for sure."

"Surgery!" the son exclaimed. Clearly, he was alarmed at the thought—much more so than his mother. Mrs. Zusman simply listened quietly.

"Let's wait and see what the X-rays show," I said soothingly. "Then you can discuss the situation further with your mother's family doctor."

Mrs. Zusman's obstruction turned out to be a gallstone that had traveled down the small intestine to a narrow place where it had become permanently lodged. Its surgical removal terminated the problem. Unfortunately, a lot of other patients aren't that lucky. My next two weren't.

I was writing up the final orders on Mrs. Zusman's chart when the biocom went off for the first time that night: "This is City Rescue Four. Come in, Memorial Hospital. How do you read us? Over."

"This is Memorial Hospital. We read City Rescue Four loud and clear."

"Ten-four, Memorial. We are at the scene with a fifty-nine-year-old woman who developed sudden severe epigastric pain and collapsed. She is alert now and says she has been having recurrent indigestion, which she has relieved by taking antacids. However, she's been under stress lately, and the pain has become worse. Initially the pain was only in the epigastric and midabdominal regions, but now she says it hurts throughout her entire abdomen."

"Any diarrhea, vomiting, or signs of hemorrhage?"

"Negative, Memorial."

"Does she hurt anyplace else?"

"Her right shoulder is hurting now. She appears to be in acute distress and extreme pain. Her pressure is one hundred over sixty. Her pulse is 130 and thready. Her respirations are twenty-eight and shallow."

"Are her lungs clear? What does her abdomen feel like?"

"The breath sounds are clear. The abdomen is very tender and rigid. It almost feels like a board."

"Okay, Rescue Four. Start an IV of normal saline and run in 500 cc's as fast as possible to get her pressure back up. Transport her Code Three."

"City Four to Memorial, we copy. This woman seems to be in a lot of pain. Should we give her some morphine?"

"That's negative on the morphine. I want to examine her first."

"Ten-four, Memorial. This is City Rescue out."

I know it must seem that the humane thing to do would be to lessen the patient's agony by giving a narcotic such as morphine. However, doing so might prove to be a fatal mistake. Morphine should never be given until it has been decided whether or not surgery will take place or until a reasonable diagnosis has been made. Morphine does little to stop serious intra-abdominal disease and can put a deceptive screen in front of the symptoms. If morphine is administered too soon, a patient may die happy with the belief that he is on the road to recovery. The hospital staff may even share this delusion. There's an old saying in medicine, "No one ever dies from pain."

If the paramedics were to sedate the woman before they brought her in, she wouldn't be able to respond clearly to my questions when I examined her, nor would she be able to give her "informed" consent for any tests or surgery I might deem necessary. I know it makes the situation difficult for the paramedics, who are on the scene and see the patient suffering but cannot give any medication without the approval of the EM physician. I'm sure that sometimes they feel resentment when they picture me sitting in a comfortable chair in front of the biocom, too far from the action to comprehend what is going on. But I am the one who is responsible for the patient, and any decision I make is based on my awareness of that responsibility.

When the paramedics arrived with the woman, her abdomen was indeed rigid and boardlike. Acid leaking out from an ulcer had caused the abdominal muscles to go into spasm. We put a tube down her stomach to drain off the acid and to check for bleeding from the ulcer.

An X-ray of her abdomen revealed air under her diaphragm. There should never be any air in the abdomen except what is enclosed in the gastrointestinal tract. Free air means there is a leak in the gastrointestinal tract. In this instance, the woman's ulcer had eaten its way through the intestinal wall. She was taken directly to surgery, and the parts of her stomach and small intestine that produce most of the acid were removed.

By the time I finished with the lady's ulcer, two more patients were waiting to see me. One was an elderly woman with abdominal pain. The other was Willie Wilson, a forty-nine-year-old alcoholic whom I see on the average of two times a month. He has virtually made me his general practitioner. I suspect this kind of relationship exists between a lot of EM physicians and certain patients who simply have nowhere else to go.

A glance at both charts indicated neither of them had acute symptoms, so I flipped a coin. The lady won.

She was sitting up on bed 6, her hands clasped across her stomach, when I stepped around the curtain. I thought she looked a lot older than the age stated on her chart: forty-seven.

"Mrs. Kott?"

She nodded.

"What's troubling you?"

"It's my appendix, Doctor. I just know it's my appendix."

"Any vomiting?" I asked.

"No, just nausea. And for the past three months, I've had constipation, then diarrhea; constipation, then diarrhea."

"Have you been losing weight?"

She nodded. "Twenty pounds in the past six weeks—and I haven't even been dieting."

"Okay. If you'll lie down, I want to feel your abdomen. After that, I'll want to get some blood tests, a stool specimen, and take some X-rays."

Her abdomen was distended and slightly tender. It was tympanitic to percussion and her bowel sounds were active. I felt no masses during abdominal or rectal examination, but her stool showed some occult blood (blood that is present in minute quantities). As little as one-half of a teaspoon of digested blood can be detected in a stool by a guaiac test. A small amount of fecal material is spread on special paper, and chemicals are added that will cause the paper to turn blue if blood is present. The occult blood in Mrs. Kott's stool was not a good sign.

Her hematocrit was 29 percent, indicating anemia, probably secondary to a small amount of bleeding from the rectum each day. And X-rays of her abdomen revealed a large-bowel obstruction.

Thirty to 40 percent of all large-bowel cancers can be felt by a simple rectal examination, and every adult over age forty should have one done as part of an annual physical examination. Blood in the stool, anemia, constipation and/or diarrhea, abdominal pain, and weight loss are all symptoms of cancer of the large bowel or colon. As the intestinal contents pass from the right side of the body to the left side, water is absorbed and the stool forms and becomes firm. Cancer of the right colon rarely obstructs, because the contents on that side are still liquid; in cancer of the left colon, obstruction dominates the picture.

I asked Mrs. Kott why she hadn't gone to see her own doctor at some point during the past six weeks.

She shrugged nervously. "I kept thinking I would. Every night when I went to bed, I'd tell myself, 'I'm going to go see Dr. Nelson tomorrow.' And then every morning when the sun came up, I'd say, 'Today's going to be better, you wait and see; today is going to be better.' But tonight the pain got so bad, I just knew tomorrow wasn't going to be any better."

I understood perfectly. "Well, I'm going to call Dr. Nelson now, Mrs. Kott. I expect the first thing he'll want is a barium enema."

She grimaced. "That sounds terrible. What is it?"

"It's just about as bad as it sounds," I said. "Barium is a white liquid that shows up well on an X-ray. It's put into an enema solution and passed up into the rectum until it fills the large intestine. The intestinal outline then shows up on the X-ray. If we were interested in the upper, or small, intestine, we'd have you *swallow* the barium, and take X-rays as it passed through the gastrointestinal tract."

I was right. Dr. Nelson did want a barium enema. While Shirley and Gloria were getting her ready, I started up the corridor to see my friend Willie Wilson, but on the way Alice nabbed me to tell me she had Dr. Kramer on the phone.

"Who's Dr. Kramer?" I asked.

"Mary McGuire's doctor," she said with a reproachful look.

"Just testing you, Alice, just testing you," I said as I picked up the receiver. "Dr. Kramer, I'm calling about a patient of yours, Mary McGuire. She had a bad fall and has four displaced fractured ribs over her liver. Her pressure is around 100 over 70 and her hematocrit is 32 percent, so she may be hemorrhaging. I feel it's advisable to admit her here since it's too dangerous to transfer her across town. I'd like to get a liver scan, and I feel we need to obtain a surgical consult as soon as possible. Do you work with anyone on staff here?"

Dr. Kramer knew one of the staff surgeons, a Dr. Hoffman, and said he'd contact him. He also okayed the liver scan. For a liver scan, the patient is injected with a radioactive isotope, which circulates throughout the body and is picked up by the liver. An X-ray is then taken, revealing the outline of the liver. Mary's liver showed a filling defect, indicating possible bleeding due to a puncture by the ribs. Grudgingly she consented to be taken to surgery. When Dr. Hoffman operated, he found more than a quart of blood enclosed in the tough fibrous capsule surrounding the liver. Fortunately, the blood hadn't broken through the capsule.

When I hung up the phone after talking to Dr. Kramer, I went to see Willie Wilson. I was a little surprised to find him alone. He's usually brought in by the police to be examined before they take him to the county jail to be "dried out." This is known as the "revolving door" system. The drunks are picked up at night and let out in the morning. The same drunks go in night after night, with no attempt made at rehabilitation.

"Hi, Willie. Where are your friends?"

He looked at me suspiciously. "Which ones?"

"The police."

"Hell, they ain't no friends of mine. All they ever do is arrest me."

"So what's your problem today?"

"Been vomiting up blood, Doc."

"How much?"

"Two—maybe three mouthfuls."

"What about your stools?"

"Stools?" He looked puzzled. I realized the only kind of stool he was familiar with was a bar stool.

"Bowel movements," I amended.

"What about 'em?"
"Have they been normal in color?"
"Nope. Dark."
"Any belly pain?"
"Yep."
"Does eating make the pain go away?"
"Yep. And drinking makes it worse."
"So why don't you stop?"
"It's the devil, Doc. I swear to God, it's the devil makes me drink."

"Yeah, well, devil or not, here's what I have to do. I need to start an IV so we can give you some fluid to replace the blood you've lost. We need to draw some blood for tests. And I'm going to put a rubber tube up your nose and down into your stomach to see if you're still bleeding, and if so, how much."

"Aw, Doc," he said. "Not that again."

"Yes, that again," I said. "If you're going to do what the devil tells you, then you're going to have to pay the price."

A patient who is vomiting blood can be a real diagnostic problem. Many of these patients are alcoholics who are brought in drunk, uncooperative, difficult to examine, stinking of booze . . . they could be bleeding from any number of places. Common symptoms of upper-gastrointestinal-tract bleeding are vague pains, a dark stool, feelings of weakness, and bloody vomitus. Swallowed blood acts as a cathartic, causing diarrhea. Blood that passes through the gastrointestinal tract and out the rectum looks tarry, black, greasy, and is foul smelling. Blood that stays in the stomach and is then vomited up looks like coffee grounds. With gastrointestinal bleeders, my job is to stabilize their blood pressure and estimate the extent of blood loss. If the bleeding is massive and can't be stopped, the patient must go straight to surgery.

Willie's history suggested either an ulcer or varicose veins in the esophagus that were oozing. Since he continued to bleed, he was taken to the operating room for surgery. It turned out to be an ulcer, and the section of his small intestine containing the ulcer was removed.

While Willie was in surgery, the X-rays from Mrs. Kott's

barium enema arrived. They showed a mass the size of a baseball blocking the large bowel. The mass, as I suspected, turned out to be cancer. I wish her diagnosis had been correct instead of mine, and it had turned out to be appendicitis.

It was getting to be around 3 A.M. Normally on a weeknight things either quiet down by then or they get weird. When I saw Shirley peering out from around the green curtain surrounding bed 5, her face verging on the color of tomato juice, I figured the latter was about to happen. She beckoned to me urgently, and I hurried over.

"What is it?" I asked her.

She handed me the chart and pointed to the place where Alice had typed: "Patient states he has something up his rectum."

Keeping my face as solemn as I could, I said, "So what's in there?"

"He thinks it's some kind of vegetable," she whispered.

"Why are you whispering?" I asked her.

"Because I . . ." she whispered, then switched to her normal voice. "I'm not."

"Six months from now, Shirley," I said, "if you're still in the emergency room, nothing will make you whisper—or blush. Believe me."

The look she gave me was one of doubt.

I walked behind the green curtain, trying to keep a straight face. I must not have succeeded, because the patient, whose name was Mr. Jarrow, said defensively, "You wouldn't laugh if it was up your ass."

I didn't bother to respond to that. "My nurse said you think it's some kind of vegetable?"

He nodded.

"Well, that won't show up on an X-ray, so I'm going to have to take a look."

I stuck my head back around the curtain and called, "Would someone step in here and help me for a minute?" All I saw of Shirley was her back as she walked quickly in the opposite direction. But Mark was coming.

I said to Mr. Jarrow, "Hop up on this surgical table, and we'll fold it up to get you in the best position. I need your buttocks sticking up in the air and your head down. Your weight should rest on your knees and elbows."

Mr. Jarrow smiled as he assumed the position I had asked for. "You won't take advantage of me, will you, Doctor?"

I ignored that, determined to be professional no matter what. "I'm going to drape some sheets over you so only your buttocks will be exposed. And then I'm going to put on a lubricated glove and see if I can feel anything in your rectum."

I couldn't feel anything with my finger, so I asked Mark for a sigmoidoscope. This is a stainless-steel tube, one inch in diameter and fifteen inches long, which is used to examine the rectum. The end of the tube that is inserted into the rectum has a light. There is a glass porthole at the other end, which is what I look through. The porthole can be opened for a biopsy to be done or to allow for suction. The rectum, the lower foot or so of the large intestine, is shaped like a lazy S. To facilitate its passage, the sigmoidoscope introduces air into the bowel, pushing the sides of the bowel away from the advancing tube. The tube is inserted past the strong anal sphincter muscles, then advanced very slowly and carefully.

No one likes to do these exams, because the porthole must be constantly opened to suction out loose fecal material. And whenever the porthole is open, gas is expelled right in the examiner's face.

"Mr. Jarrow," I said, "this isn't going to be painful, but it is going to be uncomfortable. You will feel the urge to have an enormous bowel movement. Just relax as much as possible, and try to think about something else."

I advanced the tube slowly and cautiously, inch by inch, stopping often to suction out fecal material. Five inches. Six inches. The patient didn't seem to be minding it too much. At the seven-inch mark on the sigmoidoscope, I saw a large green object. I had to look twice before I recognized what it was.

"For chrissake!" I exclaimed. "It's a cucumber."

"That bastard! Is that what he used? Wait till I get him!"

"Mark," I said, "get me those long forceps that fit down the sigmoidoscope, and I'll try to tease it out."

I tried, but every time I got hold of the cucumber with the

forceps, a small piece would break off. Pretty soon I had a small pile of cucumber pieces off to one side. I couldn't pull the cucumber out because suction was created behind it each time I tugged on it. Eventually I had to give up.

"I can't pull it out."

"But what am I going to do?"

"Well, I'll tell you. We'll give you a high retention oil enema, and you see if you can push it out on your own by morning. You know the saying, 'Whatever goes up must come down'? Well, whatever goes in must come out. If it isn't out by morning, then come back."

The cucumber wasn't the only vegetable I'd taken out of somebody's behind. One young man comes in at least once a year with a carrot embedded in him, and I've also encountered apples. Vibrators are such regular items I hardly blink. In fact, I've been considering writing the manufacturer to suggest that they attach a string for easy retrieval. Light bulbs, glasses, and Coke bottles present a little more of a challenge. Once a Coke bottle showed up on an X-ray, and I could read: "It's the real thing."

Sexual recreation does seem to bring out strange behavior patterns in people. One day last week we started out the morning with an attractive blonde woman who had apparently spent the night doing strenuous nocturnal exercises in a sports car, and her index finger had somehow gotten stuck in one of the holes in the steering wheel. She and her boyfriend tried oil, petroleum jelly, and even grease from the engine, but everything they tried only made her finger swell up more. Finally the boyfriend walked home and got some tools to detach the steering wheel from the car. When they came into the emergency room, I sent for the hospital's maintenance man; he arrived within two minutes.

"What's the problem?"

I showed him the steering wheel and asked, "Do you have anything that can cut this off, without cutting off her finger along with it?"

"I think a heavy set of wire cutters should do the trick."

Fortunately he was right. He was able to cut off two pieces from the steering wheel so the woman could remove her finger, which was a little red and sore, but intact.

One of my most memorable emergencies was Corky. When Corky's roommate was returning after a lovers' quarrel, Corky decided to meet him at the airport and surprise him with a diamond ring . . . which he slipped around his penis. Everything was all right until Corky got excited. His penis started swelling up as the blood flowed in, but the ring kept the blood from returning, and it got stuck around a sizable erection. The more Corky tried to get the ring off, the tighter the ring became.

Ultimately, Corky arrived at the emergency room. By that time his glans was swollen, tender, and purple. His problem was quickly solved when I took a ring cutter and sawed off the ring.

Thinking about Corky makes me remember the man who came in complaining of pain and swelling at the base of his penis. "I've been having vigorous sex with my girlfriend all night," he announced proudly while his hands clutched his organ very tightly.

"Please relax your hand so I can see what the problem is," I told him.

"It hurts!"

Slowly I pried his fingers from his penis long enough to take a look. Sure enough, the base was swollen and very tender. I carefully spread apart the skin and hair and saw a bright red band. At first it appeared to be blood. "My God," I thought, "he's ruptured the shaft!" But as I parted the skin and hair and looked more closely, I found a small thick red rubber band. I took a pair of curved scissors, cut it, and at once I could see his pain was relieved. "What did you do?" he asked incredulously. I held up the rubber band for him to see. He zipped up his fly, stood up, and limped out, muttering, "I'm going to kill her; so help me, I'm going to kill her."

Sometimes, of course, the things people do to themselves aren't even remotely funny. A young woman came in one time, very embarrassed, with a story about sitting on a perfume bottle. The bottle came out, but the cap got stuck and tore a hole in the side of her rectum. When I removed the cap, the blood just poured out, and she had to be taken to surgery to have the tear repaired.

I've also seen hemorrhoids and hernias bring out strange behavior patterns.

Hemorrhoids are dilated or swollen veins in the anus. Initially the treatment for hemorrhoids is conservative: stool softeners, hot tub baths, lubricants, and steroids are recommended. If this doesn't work, more rigorous methods are used, such as injecting them with phenol, or with liquid nitrogen to freeze them. Surgery is a last resort—and the only real cure.

One old codger tried to push his hemorrhoids back into his anus with a broom handle after they popped out. When that didn't work, he came to the emergency room late one night and told me to "put 'em back in."

A hernia is any abnormal opening in the abdominal wall. The most common type in men is an inguinal hernia, a weakness near where the testicles go into the abdomen. Women tend to get femoral hernias in the groin area, and in children umbilical hernias are fairly common. Hernias are dangerous only if they become strangulated—if a loop of bowel is pushed through the hernia by coughing or straining and gets stuck in such a way that the blood supply is cut off and gangrene sets in. Large hernias usually present no strangulation problem since the bowel can slip in and out easily without getting caught.

I have one patient with a huge hernia who has been coming to this emergency room as long as I've been here. He has a scrotal mass the size of a volleyball that hangs halfway down to his knees. His intestines have slipped from his abdominal cavity down through the weakness in the belly wall into the scrotal sac, and it gives him the appearance of having enormous testicles. For years I've been trying to convince him to have an operation, but he says, "Hell, no. I've got the biggest balls in town!"

These are the kinds of episodes that led me to tell Shirley that given a few more months in the emergency room, she'd forget how to blush.

I certainly remember the time I had the reddest face in town. It happened (not surprisingly) around 3 A.M. A twenty-one-year-old woman came in accompanied by her mother, who was screaming hysterically, "She's having a baby! She's having a baby!" I went out to the waiting room to tell the woman to quiet down, and I asked the daughter how many months pregnant she was.

"About seven months."

"When did you start having contractions?"

"About an hour ago. Oh, I feel another one coming on. They're getting closer together."

I scooted a nearby wheelchair under her, and after a minute she relaxed.

"If you're only seven months pregnant, and your contractions just started an hour ago," I told her, "we have plenty of time. After the clerk fills out your admission forms, we'll put you in the examination room."

She shook her head. "This is my fourth baby, Doctor. All my others came real quick."

"Did you break your water bag yet?"

"Here I go again!"

As her face twisted in pain, I undid the front of her robe and felt her abdomen. She was pregnant all right, but she felt more like eight or nine months than seven months.

Suddenly she lifted herself up on the handles of the wheelchair and started grunting and pushing.

"Don't! Don't push!" I yelled. "Wait until we get you up on a table!"

"I can't help it!"

Water mixed with mucus and blood started pouring out onto the canvas seat of the wheelchair and then the floor.

"Will you at least sit down so I can wheel you over to the delivery room? You don't want to have your baby here in the waiting room, do you?"

"It's come! It's come! It's come!"

"Sit down! Sit down! Sit down!"

The mother, by this time, was screaming, "Help her, somebody! Help her!"

I lifted up her robe. Seeing nothing, I started trying to push her back down into the wheelchair so we could get her into a private room. But her arms were locked at the elbows so I could neither push her down nor move the wheelchair.

Now she was moaning, "It came, it came, it came."

Finally I lifted up her nightgown and my eyes almost jumped out of my head. There on the canvas wheelchair seat was a squirming baby boy—who wasn't breathing, and was turning blue.

"Get me a gurney!" I yelled.

When it was brought seconds later, I tried to help her climb up onto it. A nurse was holding the wheelchair steady, but the damn gurney didn't have the brakes on, and it started to roll away from the wheelchair. The afterbirth was still attached inside the mother, and the umbilical cord was still attached to the baby. The young woman panicked and scratched and clawed her way half onto the gurney. In the process the umbilical cord twisted around her left leg and became stretched as tight as a violin string, with the baby at the other end. I picked up the baby while the nurse held the gurney steady and untwisted the cord from around the mother's leg. Finally I was able to cut the cord and suction out the baby's air passages. At last the infant took a couple of deep breaths and started crying. I put him in an incubator and was able to deliver the placenta about ten minutes later, without difficulty.

Mother and child ended up doing well. That was my first, and I hope my last, "wheelchair delivery."

7

Bystander Be Ready

I THOUGHT IT WAS going to be a run-of-the-mill Tuesday when I got to work that morning. Tuesdays, for some reason, are usually uneventful. The carryover of weekend crises dissipates on Mondays. The typical doctor's midweek holiday is on Wednesday, so we're always busy on Wednesdays. But Tuesdays are generally calm and quiet in the emergency room.

Mark and Gloria were already there when I arrived, engaged in a friendly argument about the merits of Ding Dongs versus Twinkies.

Alice greeted me with a smile, and I was scanning the charts of the two patients left over from the previous doctor's shift, as well as one who had just arrived: a little girl with a sore throat. I was letting myself anticipate a normal Tuesday, an "easy" day, when Shirley marched in. She stormed past me into the nurses' room, and I heard her bang the sliding door when she hung up her coat. Was this our Shirley of the laughing eyes? The blush that surprised nobody but her when it pinked her face the shade of Mother's Day carnations? She came out of the nurses' room with fire in her eye.

"Good lord," I exclaimed. "What happened?"

"Nothing happened," she snapped. "Absolutely nothing. That's one of life's little problems, you see. Nothing ever happens."

"If you'll give me some clue as to what you're talking about," I said, "I'll try and tune in to your wave length."

"I doubt that would be possible," she said, tossing her blond hair over her shoulder. "I just doubt that very much."

And then I remembered. On Monday nights, Shirley and a group of other nurses had recently begun attending consciousness-raising meetings.

Mark and Gloria were staring at her by then, and she glared right back at them. Especially at Gloria. "*You* should have been where I was last night," she said grimly. It was practically an accusation.

Then she turned to Mark. "And you," she said. "You'd better watch out. You know who the next black-belt champion is going to be around here?"

Mark just gaped at her helplessly, and I knew exactly how he felt.

All of our attention was abruptly switched off Shirley when Alice hurried in, saying in a strained voice, "Dr. Sword, I have a boy with a breathing problem."

Instantly, Shirley's problem was forgotten by all of us, including Shirley.

Mark grabbed a wheelchair and headed for the waiting room. Seconds later, he wheeled a teenage boy into the emergency room. I'd seen David before. He was an asthmatic. Now his color was poor, and his lips were pursed with the effort he was making to breathe.

"Let's get him on bed four," I said.

I watched as Gloria helped the boy get his shirt off. He had a barrellike chest. Air was trapped inside his lungs due to the collapsing of the small air passages and the spasms of the surrounding muscles. The air-trapping overinflates the lungs, and this is what causes the barrellike chest that is seen in people suffering from chronic obstructive lung diseases such as emphysema, and in asthmatics.

"Give him some oxygen," I said.

"Four liters per minute?" Gloria asked. She'd worked on David before, too.

I nodded.

David was having so much difficulty breathing, I doubted if he'd be able to talk very much, but I needed some answers.

"When did this attack start, David?"

"Today." He could only speak in short phrases, panting between each attempt. "This morning. . . . Been coming on . . . for days."

"What medicine have you taken within the last six hours?"

"Some aminophylline . . . but I vomited . . . it all up . . . so I used . . . the Medihaler."

Well, that was enough to get me started. I told Gloria to give him .4 cc of adrenalin, and after that to start an IV with 250 milligrams of aminophylline run in over a twenty-minute period. The oxygen was already helping him a little.

You can deprive people of food for months, and they will survive. You can deprive them of water for days, and they will survive. But if you deprive them of air for only a few minutes, they will die. Difficulty in breathing, when it's due to an airway obstruction, represents an extremely grave medical emergency—one that is more apt to involve the bystander than any other. Consequently, I feel it is absolutely essential for the general public to make itself aware of the emergency maneuvers that are necessary to establish a clear airway. If a clear airway cannot be established within minutes after an obstruction occurs, death will ensue before the victim can get to an emergency room.

Three factors must be taken into consideration when determining the degree of seriousness of an airway obstruction: the location of the obstruction, the degree of the obstruction, and the rapidity with which the obstruction develops.

An airway obstruction can be either *upper* (above the branching of the trachea, or windpipe, into the right and left main-stem bronchi) or *lower*. Lower airway obstructions are not as life threatening, because while they block some airways, they leave others open.

The most common upper airway obstruction is caused by the tongue when the patient is unconscious. As I stated in Chapter 4, the tongue, which is a muscle, relaxes and falls backward into the throat when a person is unconscious.

Other common causes of upper airway obstruction include severe tonsillitis, vomitus, dentures, small toys children put in their mouths, and food.

The term "cafe coronary" is used to describe an upper airway obstruction caused by the inhalation of a large piece of food. When an overweight middle-aged male who is in a restaurant drinking and eating too much and too fast suddenly collapses, the people nearby will assume the man is having a heart attack, and someone will summon an ambulance. But if a person—*any* person—suddenly collapses while eating, nine times out of ten it is not a heart attack, but a large piece of food lodged in the throat. Often people who have inhaled a piece of food, out of fear of embarrassment, will leave the table and lock themselves in the bathroom while they try to dislodge it by coughing. And not infrequently they will end up dead on the bathroom floor before anyone even realizes what has happened.

An important point to remember is that normal breathing is effortless and silent. In either upper or lower airway obstruction, the breathing will become noisy and labored. The victim of an obstructed upper airway will have a sudden onset of labored breathing with a tremendous inspiratory effort. He may become blue, and his lips and/or eyes may bulge as he tries to take in air. Coughing or talking becomes impossible. Ultimately the effort to breathe will cease, and the victim will collapse.

Whoever is at the scene *must*—I repeat, *must*—find a way to open the victim's airway. Often, as I mentioned in Chapter 4, this may be accomplished, with the patient lying on his back, by hyperextending the head and neck to remove the tongue from the back of the throat. To do this the rescuer places one hand under the patient's neck and the other on the patient's forehead, lifting up on the back of the neck with one hand while at the same time applying pressure on the forehead in the opposite direction. This draws the tongue forward.

If spontaneous breathing does not occur after the head-tilt maneuver, the rescuer must bring the hand that is pressing down on the forehead farther down to close the victim's nostrils. The rescuer then blows four short breaths into the victim's mouth. If spontaneous breathing still does not occur, an immediate attempt must be made to clear the airway. The rescuer must roll the victim away from himself, then place his knee under the victim's shoulders and administer several sharp blows with the heel of the hand between the victim's shoulder blades. In young children and infants, a sharp blow to the middle of the back or a sharp squeeze of the lower chest is usually best. If you're involved in trying to clear someone's airway, don't worry about breaking a few ribs; it's a small price to pay for saving a life. An alternate technique often used effectively is the Heimlich maneuver. While standing behind the victim, the rescuer must place his arms around the victim's abdomen, interlocking his own hands together, and apply a quick squeeze (like a bear hug) with a forceful upward thrust. This technique causes a sudden elevation of the diaphragm which will sometimes jar the obstruction loose. After attempting any of these maneuvers, the rescuer should then probe the victim's mouth to determine whether any foreign objects were dislodged.

If none of these techniques has been successful, and there *is* a foreign object stuck in the throat, a tracheotomy, or a cricothyrotomy must be done. And whoever is on the scene, involved in an attempt to save the victim, must do it. It's a last resort, but the alternative is death.

A cricothyrotomy is by far the easiest. The rescuer must feel for the victim's Adam's apple. Then, using a knife or anything available that will cut, place it horizontally a finger's breadth down from the victim's Adam's apple, and cut firmly through the skin to a depth of about three-fourths of an inch. This opening may be enlarged by spreading both ends, and putting in something—a ballpoint pen, for example—to hold it open. If there's any kind of tube available, this can be put into the opening. The rescuer must then breathe directly into the opening in the throat, or through the tube which has been inserted into the throat.

In an upper airway obstruction, such as food inhalation, the primary problem is getting air *in*. In lower airway obstructions, like David's, the problem is getting the air out.

David had started to breathe easier fairly quickly, thanks to the adrenalin. Physicians have to be extremely careful when administering it, however—especially to older people or anyone with heart problems—because it can cause cardiac arrest and death.

I told Gloria to let the rest of the IV solution run in (in order to rehydrate him), and then I bent down to listen to his lungs. I could still hear some wheezing.

Wheezing is one of the characteristics of asthma. The sound is caused by a narrowing of the small airways due to spasm, a swelling of the mucous membranes, and an increase in secretions.

This becomes easier to understand if you picture the lungs as two trees hanging upside down. The "leaves" on the tree branches are called alveoli. There are 2 to 4 million alveoli. The gas exchange between oxygen and carbon dioxide takes place in the alveoli. If air cannot reach the alveoli, there can be no exchange of gases. As I mentioned in Chapter 3, the surface area of the lungs is about the size of a tennis court. The blood spends only half a second on this surface while the exchange between oxygen and carbon dioxide is taking place.

If you ever want to know what asthma feels like, bury your head in a wool blanket. You'll wheeze—which is a normal response. Asthmatics spend a large part of their lives wheezing, because they are as highly sensitive to innumerable substances and stimuli as the average person is to chlorine gas. The major problem faced by asthmatics is bronchospasm, a sharp contraction of the bronchial tubes. Fortunately, there are several medications that relieve the asthmatic's resulting shortness of breath and difficulty in breathing.

Since David was still wheezing some, I told Shirley to call Inhalation Therapy and have them give him fifteen minutes of breathing into the intermittent positive pressure breathing (IPPB) machine, using one-half cc of isoproterenol, and two cc's of saline for a breathing mist.

When the inhalation therapist arrived with the IPPB machine, he asked David if he'd been using his nebulizer too frequently.

David said, "I'm afraid so."

The inhalation therapist nodded sympathetically, saying, "Well, you really shouldn't use it too often—not over four times a day. You can't use it every time you wheeze or it loses its effectiveness, you get a rebound effect, and your wheezing becomes much worse."

"I know," David replied. "But when I can't breathe I get panicky, and I forget what I should do."

The inhalation therapist set up the IPPB machine, promising David he'd have him feeling a lot better very soon.

Which was true. David would feel better—until the next attack. There just is no real cure for severe asthmatics. I knew David's chances of having another attack during the next twenty-four hours were high, so I ordered a shot of Sus-Phrine, which is adrenalin dissolved in a glycerin base, for him before he went home. This would give him relief for up to twelve hours.

After I left David, I went to see the little girl with the sore throat. Her mother was holding a children's book in her lap, but she wasn't reading it. The child was sitting up on the edge of the bed, swinging her feet back and forth. When children are nervous they always seem to manage to keep some part of their body in motion, and often it's the feet. The little girl was probably too nervous to be read to. Hospitals can be scary places for kids. Emergency rooms must be especially frightening when children who are sick with a cold or the flu have to sit and wait, sometimes for hours, while we rush around trying to help someone who is a lot worse off than they are.

I always try to relax children. Sometimes I try so hard I suspect I look like Chuckles the Clown on TV.

"Hello," I said with a happy smile, "what's your name?"

"Charlotte," she said, in a squeaky little sore-throat voice.

"That's a nice name. And how old are you?"

"Four and a half."

"You're sure?" I said.

She nodded solemnly.

"You look more like four and five-eighths to me."

Her expression didn't change. Why should it? She didn't even know what "five-eighths" was. But her mother gave me a thanks-for-trying smile.

"How long has she been sick?" I asked.

"She hasn't been feeling well since last night. She woke up

this morning feeling hot, so I kept her home from preschool. I called her doctor, but he won't be in until tomorrow."

"Has she complained of anything herself?"

"She said her head and stomach and throat hurt."

I checked her ears, nose, throat, neck, heart, lungs, stomach, and joints. I found nothing obvious but a runny nose.

"No vomiting, diarrhea, coughing, or pain with urination?" I asked.

"I don't think so. Does it hurt when you go to the bathroom?" asked the mother.

The little girl shook her head.

"Probably she just has a virus or a cold," I said. "But I'll culture her throat for beta strep anyway. It takes two days to grow out the bacteria from the culture. Meanwhile, see that she gets plenty of rest and give her lots of fluids. You may give her four baby aspirin or one adult aspirin."

The mother looked surprised. "An adult aspirin? Isn't she too young?"

"The dosage is generally one baby aspirin for each year of life until the age of four or five. Four baby aspirin, you see, equal one adult aspirin. I'll also give you a prescription for some antihistamine to dry up her nose."

"Aren't you going to give her a shot for her sore throat?"

I shook my head. In children, 90 percent of sore throats are caused by a virus, and viruses aren't affected by antibiotics. It's impossible to tell just by looking whether a sore throat is being caused by strep or by a virus. Lay people use the term *strep* to mean any bad sore throat. Most viruses will cause a sore throat for only a limited period of time. The virus-caused sore throat will get better in two to five days' time whether or not antibiotics are used. So a patient whose throat isn't getting better by the second or third day will go and see his doctor and insist on having a shot, and lo and behold, the sore throat goes away in one or two days' time. What the patient doesn't understand is that the sore throat would have burned itself out anyway in the same length of time. Strep lasts about the same length of time as a virus infection. What is different about strep, and the reason we treat it with so much respect, is the aftermath of rheumatic fever that can occur following a strep infection. This happens in 3 to 5 percent of people who have a strep throat, but it can be totally prevented by penicillin. Taking time to do a throat culture before administering antibiotics has been shown not to cause any increase in rheumatic fever.

Giving antibiotics unnecessarily, however, is something I try hard not to do. Not only will antibiotics have no effect on viruses, but they can cause allergic reactions and even death. If an antibiotic is used frivolously, when we really need to use it, the patient may have developed an allergy to it. Ten to 15 percent of children today are already allergic to penicillin, which is our best antibiotic. In addition, antibiotics tend to lose their effectiveness as bacteria adapt to them. Many bacteria used to be so sensitive to penicillin that a shot of only 10,000 units would produce a cure. Now the same kinds of bacteria need a shot of 4,800,000 units to produce a cure, or almost 500 times as much. And the recommended dosage goes up every year.

Bacteria other than strep aren't affected very much by penicillin, so we have to use more toxic (to humans) and less effective antibiotics to kill them. The question of if, when, and which antibiotics are to be given is an area of constant active debate among physicians.

Unfortunately, many parents take their children to the doctor at the first sign of sickness and demand a shot. Rather than patiently explaining the pros and cons of injecting penicillin, the doctor frequently finds it less time-consuming to just give the shot. It's what people have come to expect: something for their money. For some people, that old bromide, "If it hurts it must be good," still carries weight.

I took a few minutes to explain all this to Charlotte's mother, and when I finished, she simply said, "You'll call me, then, if her culture yields strep?"

"We'll call and tell you either way," I assured her.

As I walked out to the admitting desk to finish writing on Charlotte's chart, Alice told me that she had put a penis problem in our private examining room.

I stopped writing and looked at her. "A penis problem?"

She nodded matter-of-factly.

"What kind of a penis problem?"

"Oh, you know," she said, and waved her hand airily. "The usual."

"Oh," I said.

I finished Charlotte's chart and walked around the corner into our private examining room, wondering just what our "usual" penis problem was. A thin, balding man I judged to be in his late thirties was sitting up gingerly on the edge of the bed.

"Hi," I said. "What's the problem?"

He looked worriedly over the top of his thick-lensed glasses at me. "When I got up this morning, I had this erection. It's happened before, and it's never bothered me. I . . . uh . . . live alone. Usually I just urinate and it goes right down, but this time it didn't. It's still as hard as a rock. At first I thought it was kind of funny. There's this woman, Irma, whose desk is right across from mine in the insurance office where I work. I sit and stare at her legs all day long. I mean, every time I look up from my work, they're there, you know? And I thought to myself, gee, maybe I should call up Irma. But after it started to hurt, it wasn't funny anymore. What's the matter with me? Am I oversexed?"

He asked this last question in a tone that might be construed as hopeful.

"No," I said. "What's happening to you is called priapism. It's caused by the blood becoming so thick that it's unable to leave your penis, resulting in a prolonged erection."

"But why? What causes it to happen? It isn't because I sit and stare at Irma's legs all day, is it?"

"I doubt it," I said, trying not to smile. "A lot of cases are associated with sickle cell anemia or leukemia. I'll order some blood tests in order to rule those out. In the meantime, we'll give you an ice-water enema."

"A *what?*"

"An ice-water enema," I repeated. "Unfortunately, with priapism your chances of becoming impotent increase the longer the condition is allowed to go untreated. If the enema doesn't work, I'll have to call a urologist and have him evacuate the sludged blood from your penis with a needle and syringe."

"Oh, lord," he said.

"Why don't you lie down," I suggested.

He did, without another word. As I was leaving the room, I heard him murmur softly, "I promise I'll never look at Irma's legs again."

I intended to tell Mark to give the poor man his cold-water enema, but as I headed down the corridor looking for him, Alice flagged me down to tell me that Hermosa Beach Rescue was bringing in a "near drowning," and that Mark was preparing bed 4. Shirley happened to be dead center in my line of vision right then, so I said, "Shirley, would you give the man in our examining room a cold-water enema?"

Shirley glared at me with iceberg eyes, then spun around on her heel and marched off to do what I'd told her.

I might have followed her to ask just what the hell was going on with her this morning, but the Hermosa Beach paramedics arrived at that particular moment and I didn't have time.

They wheeled in a wan-faced teenage girl, her light brown hair plastered in wet curls against her skull. Her eyes were closed, but she seemed to be breathing okay.

"She's not too bad," one of the paramedics told me. "She never lost consciousness. But the life guards said she swallowed a lot of water. Her pulse and blood pressure are good, and she'll answer you if you shake her hard."

"How old is she?"

"She says sixteen, but I'd guess fourteen tops."

"Anybody with her?"

He shook his head.

The girl was our fourth near-drowning this week. An article I'd read the week before stated that drowning was the second leading cause of death in people under age twenty-four (the first was auto accidents); that four out of five drowning victims were male; and that one out of three were people who knew how to swim.

An interesting fact that many people are unaware of is that humans are born with what might be termed an "antidrowning" reflex. When babies up to the age of four months are placed prone in the water with their faces submerged, they exhibit a marked swimming reflex—a definite rhythmic action, not only in the arms and legs but also from side to side in the torso. These movements are in fact forceful enough to propel the baby a short distance through the water. In addition, newborn infants when submerged in water will—apparently through a reflex that inhibits breathing while submerged—control their breathing. And the swimming motions they make while controlling their breathing become stronger and more pronounced. Unfortunately, after about the age of four months these helpful reflexes tend to weaken, and older humans in trouble in the water cough and thrash and struggle and do everything they shouldn't do.

The majority of people I talk to believe that getting salt water in your lungs is twice as bad as getting fresh water. Actually, it's half a dozen of one and six of the other. Salt water is four times saltier than blood, so when you get salt water in your lungs, plasma floods in trying to dilute it, which only makes it worse. The result is called pulmonary edema. If a lot of plasma goes into your lungs, the blood pressure drops off and shock develops. With fresh water, half the water inhaled is absorbed by the lungs in one to three minutes. (That's why it's almost useless to turn people over to try to drain the water out of them.) The fresh water itself damages the delicate little blood vessels in the lungs, causing plasma to leak out and resulting in the same flooding of the lungs—pulmonary edema—as with salt water. So whether a near-drowning occurs in fresh or salt water, the end result is the same, and so is the treatment. What we try to do is correct the primary consequence, which is hypoxemia, or lack of oxygen in the blood.

As the paramedics moved the girl from their gurney up onto bed 4, her eyelids fluttered and then she opened her eyes. I bent down to listen to her lungs, which sounded all right.

She gave me a tremulous smile that made her look about ten years old. She seemed very fragile to me, very vulnerable.

"What's your name?" I asked her.

"Sarah," she answered.

"Do you remember what happened?"

"Not too much. I was swimming, and a big wave came in when I wasn't looking, and knocked me down. And then there were just a whole lot of people around."

"What were you looking at instead of the wave?" I asked her.

She gave a funny little shrug and sighed. "The life guard. That's why I've been going to the beach so early in the morning. It's the only time I figured he might . . . well, you know, notice me."

I nodded. "I bet he noticed you today."

"I guess so. There were so many people around me, I didn't even see whether he was one of them."

"How do you feel now?"

"Scared."

"Well, look, Sarah," I said. "You seem to be all right. We'll get a chest X-ray and some blood gases to make sure, and if everything checks out, I'll send you home. Okay?"

"Ye-es," she said. "Except nobody's home. My mom works, and I sort of don't feel like being alone. Could I just stay here a while?"

"It'll take a while to get your tests done," I said. "But is there someone we can call who would come and stay with you? We can call your mother at work."

"No, she'd be real mad at me. My brother, maybe. He wouldn't mind. He loves to get called away from work."

"Brother it is, then. And listen."

"Hm?"

"Next time, watch the waves."

As I left the cubicle where Sarah was, I almost collided with Shirley, marching down the corridor in the opposite direction.

"The cold-water enema didn't work, Dr. Sword," she snapped.

"Then get the on-call urologist down here," I snapped right back. "And after you've done that, come into the doctor's room and give me a fast five minutes of your time."

I finished writing on Sarah's chart, got two cartons of orange juice out of the refrigerator, and went to the doctor's room to wait for Shirley. When she came, she marched into the room and then stood in front of me as if I had said "A-ten-shun!"

"Hey," I said. "Truce." And I held out the carton of orange juice.

She took it, and started to unbend. A little.

I gestured toward an empty chair.

She looked at it skeptically, but finally she sat down.
Then I said, "What's wrong?"
"I hate to give enemas," she snapped.
"Sure," I replied. "Everybody does. So what else is wrong?"
"I just didn't know enough about the kind of work nurses have to do," she said. "I thought it was going to be different."

I know that happens to lots of people who go into nursing. Books, movies, and television project a fairy-tale image of the profession. The reality is that nurses take care of sick people, who vomit, have diarrhea in their beds, cough up yellow smelly sputum, leak urine around their catheters and all over their bedclothes. They have bed sores and dressings full of pus and blood that need to be changed. Sick people are sick people, not the glamorous languishing invalids you see on daytime soap operas. So anybody, male or female, who is thinking about going into nursing should spend some time at a garden-variety local hospital with the line nurses before making up his or her mind to become a nurse.

But it didn't ring true to me that the reality of nursing was what was bothering Shirley. She functioned too well and was too anxious to learn. I figured it had to be something else, maybe the pay. A starting RN gets about $16,000 a year, a supervisor $20,000 —which, as they say, "ain't much" when compared with what plumbers get. I decided to play detective.

"It's a lousy job, nursing," I said. "And the pay's bad, too."

She looked at me in surprise. Then, after a moment, she said, "That's not the worst part."

"Of course not," I agreed. "It's the damn hours. The trouble with sick people is they're sick twenty-four hours a day, day in, day out, weekends, holidays. Even on Christmas they're sick. Believe me, I know how hard nursing hours are on your personal life."

But old Sherlock Sword was wrong again.

"Even that," Shirley said ominously, "isn't the worst part."

"It isn't?"

"No. Did you know that less than fifty percent of nurses with degrees are still practicing?"

"Well, I—" But she didn't even hear me.

"And do you want to know why? I'll tell you why. Do you know what nurses do? I'll tell you what they do. They follow a doctor's orders. The doctor decides everything: what tests to order, what medicine and how much, when the patient is to be admitted and when the patient is to go home. The doctor gets all the glory and all the money, and the nurses do all the dirty work."

I really had to bite my tongue in order not to respond to her anger with anger of my own, but that wouldn't have gotten us anywhere. Since Shirley had started going to consciousness-raising meetings, she had come in boiling on a couple of Tuesdays before this one and had taken the rest of the day to simmer down. She'd been mad at automobile mechanics, truck drivers, and hard-hat construction workers. But this was the first time she'd made doctors the focus of her attack. I didn't feel it was justified.

"Hey, somebody has to be the general," I told her. "You can't have a committee taking care of a patient. And it's part of a doctor's training: A doctor is taught how to assume the burden of responsibility. I'm just not sure what you're getting at."

"What I'm getting at," she said, "is incompetent doctors."

"Like who?" I asked her.

"Like who? *Like who?* I'll tell you like who. Like the ones you talk to all the time who won't come in when you ask them to. Like the ones who aren't on call when they're supposed to be. Like the ones who shouldn't even be practicing medicine, who do substandard work and then expect their nurses to cover up for them. You should have heard some of the stories I heard last night, then you'd know what I'm talking about."

Well, I'd let off enough steam on these issues myself, so I wasn't in a position to criticize her for doing it.

"I've felt what you're feeling a lot of times," I told her. "But when I'm not angry, when I can stand back and take the long view, I can see that there is a kind of ultimate justice that dogs our system. You know, if some nurses feel there is a serious problem with the way a given doctor is practicing medicine, they can report it to the appropriate medical committee. I can name you six doctors who were on staff here last year but can no longer admit patients to this hospital. And doctors have their own ways of censuring their colleagues. If they know somebody is doing substandard work, they simply stop referring patients to him."

She looked down at her orange-juice carton and didn't say anything.

"Maybe," I said, "you ought to think about becoming a general yourself."

She looked up. "What do you mean?"

"I mean if you want more say-so, more responsibility, then equip yourself to get a position that will give it to you."

"Go to medical school, you mean?"

"Why not?"

She heaved a deep sigh. "I need to think about it," she said. "I have been, but I have to think about it some more. It's always easier to get mad about something than it is to think about it."

"I know," I said. "I do it all the time."

She gave me a small smile and stood up. "Yeah, well, I guess I'd better get back to work." She walked out of the doctor's room —which was better than marching out.

My wife, Sandra, has managed to raise my level of consciousness a few degrees. I know women face tough choices today. Medicine, for example. Once upon a time, the door was virtually shut in a woman's face. She had two choices: walk away, or try to batter the door down. Now the door is open, and women have to decide whether they want to give up four to eight years of their life, putting a career first; whether they want to combine (and are capable of combining) childbearing and child-rearing with career goals, or whether they want to forego childbearing. The decisions can't be easy.

It sure hadn't been the best day for me to tell Shirley to give a cold-water enema to a man with a permanent erection. But that is life in the emergency room.

8

A True Pandora's Box

THE BRAIN—that incredibly complex organ that harbors so many of man's mysteries: his mind, his dreams—there is no body part more frightening to attempt to treat when it's in jeopardy. The heart and the lungs have their own repertoire of terrors for the EM physician. But the head, the brain within, is the true Pandora's box.

Neolithic cave men's skulls show evidence of having been trepanned (having had holes drilled in them). Anthropologists assume this was done to let out the evil, pain-causing spirits. Drastic remedy, you think, for a headache? Read on. Sometimes we drill such holes today.

The number of things that can injure the head is, of course, legion: bullets, baseball bats, bricks, virtually any hard surface with which the head has an opportunity to come into contact—a street curb, for example.

It was a Thursday morning. I was working the 7 A.M. to 7 P.M. shift, and the emergency room was quiet. Shirley and Gloria were discussing the Mobile Intensive Care Nurses' Test they were both planning to take. Mark and Alice were trying to fill in the last half-dozen words in the daily crossword puzzle. I was sitting with my feet propped up on my desk, browsing through the current medical journals, when the familiar *ding dong* shattered the silence: "This is City Rescue One. Come in, Memorial." I went to the monitor, flipped it on, started the tape recorder, and pressed the microphone button: "This is Memorial Hospital. Go ahead, City Rescue."

"Ten-four, Memorial. We have a thirty-six-year-old male who fell off his bike when his front wheel went into the grid of a drain sewer. His wife, who was riding with him at the time, said he struck the right side of his head on the curb. He was unconscious for a minute or two and then tried to get up. She persuaded him to remain lying down, and a passerby called us. Since we arrived on the scene, he keeps trying to get up, keeps saying he's all right, and gets mad as hell when we restrain him."

I didn't like the sound of it. "Do you have vital signs?" I asked.

"Negative, but there's no breathing problem."

Damn, I wished I could be there, to see, to touch, to listen. "What's his level of consciousness? How about his pupils? Is he moving his extremities? His neck? Are there any obvious signs of injury?"

"He has a large bruise and swelling on the right side of his neck. He's moving all extremities, also his neck. He's not bleeding externally. We can't see his pupils; he's too combative."

I shook my head. "City Rescue One, you may be dealing with an epidural hemorrhage. Bring him in at once—even if you have to get the police to handcuff him. And try to start an IV of normal saline."

From the paramedic's brief description of the patient's behavior, I suspected I knew what was going on. When we sprain an ankle or break a wrist, there's plenty of space inside our skin to accommodate the swelling that occurs as a reaction to the injury. But when the brain is injured, the swelling is confined within a closed space, the skull, which causes a rise in the intracranial pressure. This results in a compression of the blood vessels, thus shutting off the supply of oxygen. Hypoxia (lack of oxygen) then causes even more swelling, which leads to an additional increase in pressure. Unless this cycle is broken rapidly, death occurs.

When the paramedics arrived a few minutes later and wheeled the patient into the critical care area, the anxiety in their faces heightened my suspicions.

A distraught young woman, her eyes huge in her pale face, was gripping the side of the gurney on which the man lay quietly.

My eyes questioned the paramedic nearest me.

"He got real lethargic all of a sudden," the paramedic said. "We didn't have to handcuff him."

"You're his wife?" I asked the woman.

She nodded jerkily.

"You'll have to wait outside."

"Oh, please, I—"

"I'm sorry," I said firmly. "I have to give my full attention to your husband. I'll come out and talk with you just as soon as I can."

As Mark and Alice led her away, the woman kept looking backward over her shoulder at me. I knew all too well what she was feeling. Every patient and every relative or friend who brings a patient to the hospital emergency room has anxiety on two levels: about the nature and severity of the illness or injury; and about what is going to happen inside the emergency room. They're dependent upon people with whom they've had no opportunity to establish a trust relationship. This woman's husband had been critically injured, and she was leaving him in the hands of a total stranger. It had to be scary as hell for her.

I looked down at the injured man. "What's his name?" I asked the paramedic.

"Ken Lane."

Leaning over the bed railing, I said, "Ken? Ken, can you hear me?" I got no response.

When a person suffering a head injury regains consciousness quickly but then lapses into lethargy (as Ken did), it's often far more serious than when a person is knocked out and then slowly regains consciousness. The latter case is probably just a concussion, while the former indicates progressively increasing intracranial pressure.

Always, with head injuries, the primary consideration is maintaining an adequate supply of oxygen. The brain is more sensitive to lack of oxygen than any organ in the body, and its tissue can't survive for more than four or five minutes without oxygen. The level of consciousness is the best indicator as to whether or not the brain is receiving enough oxygen. To determine what this level is, we find out what it takes to awaken the patient, or at least elicit some sort of response.

I put my two forefingers inside Ken Lane's clenched fists. "Ken," I said, "if you can hear me, squeeze my fingers twice."

No response.

Shaking him brusquely, I called out, "Ken, Ken, open your eyes!"

Still nothing.

Since there was no response to spoken commands, I briskly rubbed my fingers on his sternum (breastbone). This is a painful stimulus, and he didn't like it. His right hand came up defensively and pushed my knuckles away. At the same time, his right leg flexed. But his left hand hung limp, and his left leg didn't move.

Gloria, watching intently, anticipated my next move and handed me an open safety pin. When I stuck the point deeply into the soles of his feet and then the tips of his fingers, I elicited the same response: a withdrawal reaction on the right side, but no movement on the left.

Growing more concerned by the second, I checked his pupils with a flashlight beam. The left pupil reacted by constricting sharply to the light. The reaction of the right pupil, which seemed more dilated, was sluggish. There was no longer any room for doubt. I was facing a grave medical emergency: an epidural hemorrhage.

An epidural hemorrhage occurs when an artery inside the skull ruptures. This produces an expanding clot of blood between the skull bone and the dura (the tough protective membrane covering the brain). The expanding blood clot has no place to go, so the blood vessels to the brain are compressed, leading to an avalanche of events that can culminate in death. If the bleeding is from a low-pressure vessel, a vein, the avalanche takes a while to gather momentum. Blood clots from veins usually occur under the dura, hence are called "subdural" hematomas (clots). But the avalanche is rapid if the bleeding is from an artery.

With Ken Lane, I sensed the whole damn mountain about to come down on me. The atmosphere of my emergency room, which less than half an hour ago had been as quiet as a ski lodge when the first powder snow of the season is on the ground, was now charged with tension that was almost tangible. I started barking out orders like the top sergeant of a marine platoon:

"Alice, get Dr. Schepper on the line." Dr. Schepper was the staff neurosurgeon on call. "And alert the operating room that we have a priority case.

"Shirley, have the lab draw some blood for type and cross-match—six units—plus a CBC, BUN, glucose, and electrolytes. Have X-ray take portable films of his head and neck. Include a chest plate, too.

"Gloria, let's get an IV started on the left side. He won't move when you stick him there."

"What kind of fluid, and how fast do you want it run in?" she asked.

"Normal saline, and run it in at TKO [to keep open] only. After you get that started, hang a drip of mannitol at two grams per kilogram of his body weight. What do you think he weighs?"

Gloria was a genius at guessing body weight, probably because she was so sharply conscious of the fluctuations in her own.

"I'd say around one eighty."

"That's about eighty kilograms. Okay, give him one hundred sixty grams of mannitol over twenty minutes. Add twelve milligrams of Decadron as a bolus, too." A bolus means that the steroid, Decadron, is injected into the IV over seconds rather than minutes.

The mannitol would dehydrate him and shrink his brain by removing some of the water from it. By thus countering some of the pressure from the expanding blood clot in Ken Lane's head, we could buy the time we needed to get X-rays, get the blood bank ready, and assemble the operating-room crew so they'd be ready when Dr. Schepper arrived to drill the holes in the skull that would relieve the pressure, and tie off the bleeding artery.

"Do you want a Foley catheter in?" Shirley asked.

"Yes! Thank you."

I'm fortunate in having excellent nurses, who are always thinking. Good nurses are worth double, triple their weight in gold—especially to an emergency medicine physician. Elsewhere in the hospital (in the cardiac care unit, for example), nurses tend to develop in-depth relationships with patients whom they tend for days, or even weeks. In the emergency room, there isn't time for such a relationship to develop. At the most we spend only hours with a patient, and so the in-depth relationships we develop are with each other. Go through a few life-and-death encounters with someone and you soon find out what makes them tick. And they, you.

I care professionally and personally about the nurses I work with. My ego isn't threatened when they take the initiative. Indeed, when I'm trying to remember twenty-five things in fifteen seconds, I'm grateful for it. Of course the ultimate responsibility is all mine. But in spite of that, or perhaps because of it, I welcome all the help I can get.

By putting a Foley catheter in Mr. Lane, not only could we monitor his hourly urinary output (chapter 4 explained the importance of doing this), but we would also prevent his bladder from becoming distended. An unconscious patient can be made just as irritable and restless by a distended bladder as can a conscious one, and people with head injuries need to be kept as quiet as possible.

Despite everything we were doing for him, Ken Lane was lapsing into ever deeper levels of unconsciousness—which meant the carbon dioxide level in his blood was probably increasing, as was the swelling of the brain tissue. His pulse had begun to slow down, his blood pressure was climbing, and his breathing was becoming slow and labored. I told Mark to call Inhalation Therapy and tell them to come down right away, and I asked Gloria to get me the intubation tray.

I knew I either had to do a tracheostomy (open the trachea directly in order to insert a tube) or else put a nasotracheal tube in him. Usually in order to put in the latter you have to hyperextend the neck to the sniffing position, as I did with Mr. Gootee in chapter 4. However, since Mr. Lane had fallen on his head and could possibly have a broken neck with an unstable fracture, I couldn't risk moving his neck. Consequently, I wouldn't be able to see where I was going.

Physicians, like magicians, sometimes resort to trickery. In a case like this, the trick I use is to measure the distance from the tip of the patient's ear to the tip of his nose, and mark that distance on the nasotracheal tube. I then put the tube through the nose down to the mark I have made on the tube. If my patient's physiology is normal, I should be just above the epiglottis and the vocal cords. I wait for the patient to take in a breath, then I shove the tube down the windpipe. If I still hear breath sounds, I know I'm in the trachea. If the tube accidentally slides into the esophagus, all breath sounds stop, and I pull the tube back out to the mark I made, wait for the next inspiratory breath, and try again. If I have to perform this procedure on a patient who isn't breathing, after I think the tube is in the trachea I breathe into it. If it is correctly positioned, the patient's chest will rise; if it is in the esophagus, his stomach will puff up. This might all sound easy but believe me, it's not.

When the inhalation therapist arrived, I told him Mr. Lane wasn't breathing very well, so I was going to put down a nasotracheal tube.

"After I get it down," I said, "put him on the Bird machine and force-breathe him to get rid of some carbon dioxide. Then get a new set of blood gases."

"What size tube do you want?" he asked.

"Seven millimeters."

He selected the proper tube, lubricated it to make it slide down the nose easier, and handed it to me.

I slipped the eleven-inch plastic tube through Mr. Lane's nose and into his trachea in one smooth motion.

"That sure went in easy," Gloria said.

I nodded. I'd been lucky, but I wasn't through with Mr. Lane yet. I told Gloria to put a nasal-gastric tube down the other side of his nose and hook it up to low suction. This would keep his stomach empty and prevent abdominal distention.

By now my patient looked like a character in a science-fiction movie: an IV on his left side, a catheter in his penis, and tubes running out of both nostrils. I didn't care what he looked like; I just wanted him to live. But I wasn't at all certain he was going to, and I had just about run out of moves.

"Alice!" I yelled. "Did you get hold of Dr. Schepper?"

Alice hurried into the critical care area. "His answering service said he wasn't available right now, and they would call us back when he was."

"Sweet Jesus!" I barked. "That is not acceptable. Call them back right now and explain the nature and urgency of the problem. Ask them if anyone else is taking his calls—and document the number of times you talk to the answering service; write down everything they say."

She went to do what I told her. Moments later, she was back. "Dr. Schepper's line is busy," she said. "And you don't know how much I hate to tell you this, but there's an elderly man in the waiting room in a lot of pain. He says he can't urinate."

"Alice . . ." I moaned.

"He does seem to be hurting a great deal," she said.

"Okay. Mark, put the poor man in bed six, and tell him I'll get back to see him as soon as I can."

As Mark and Alice left, the X-ray technician arrived. "What pictures do you want?"

"A lateral of his head and his neck, and a chest film if you can slip the cassette under his back without moving his neck."

I moved away from Mr. Lane to give the X-ray technician more room, and nearly collided with Alice.

"I hope you're here to tell me you have Dr. Schepper on the line," I said.

She shook her head. "Every time I pick up the phone, Mrs. Lane interrupts me. Could you please, *please* come and talk to her? She's almost hysterical."

"Not now," I said. "Not yet. Try to calm her down—and keep trying to get hold of Dr. Schepper."

As she turned to go, her face was taut with frustration. I didn't have time to think about it much, because Mark was waving at me from bed 6. There wasn't anything I could do for Ken Lane at that point, so I started down the corridor toward Mark. The walk was a long one because I was thinking about Ken with each step I took. Was I doing everything possible? Was I forgetting anything? Could someone else do a better job? I was hanging self-doubts around my neck like a whole flock of albatrosses. I felt so helpless watching the man slide downhill. I knew what had to be done: The pressure inside his skull had to be relieved. What I wanted to do was haul the man into surgery, open up his head, relieve the pressure, find the bleeding artery, and tie it off. Legally all I could do was stabilize him . . . and wait.

I literally had to shake myself to attention as I drew near bed 6, where I suddenly became aware that I wasn't the only one who had to wait: An elderly man was lying there waiting patiently for *me*. His skin hung on him so loosely it looked like a shabby, too-large overcoat that had worn thin over his joints and hands; the skin there was almost transparent. His lower abdomen was round and firm like a volleyball, extending upward almost to his umbilicus. His bladder was swollen to capacity. A catheter had been inserted into his penis; the other end was attached to a plastic bag that was taped to his leg.

"Jeez, am I glad to see you, Doc. I can't piss anymore."

"You look pretty uncomfortable," I agreed. "How long has it been?"

"For the past two days, only a little piss comes out at a time, and then only if I press down on my bladder. Then it leaks out around the catheter."

"Anything else bothering you?"

"That's a long story you probably don't have the time to listen to. All I want is for you to get this damn thing working again."

"How long have you had that catheter in?" I asked him.

"About four months now."

"It's probably plugged," I said. "Catheters should be changed every one to three months, depending on the type. Don't you have a family doctor?"

"No, I just moved out here. Been putting off getting a doctor —you know how it is."

I turned to Mark. "Change his catheter, irrigate his bladder, and measure the amount of urine you get."

"Dr. Sword!"

Gloria's voice rang out from the critical care area.

"Mr. Lane is having a seizure!"

I hurried back up the corridor to the critical care area, rolled Ken Lane over onto his left side and asked grimly, "How did it start?

"First his eyes looked strongly to the left. Then his head turned to the left. At the same time, he curled up his right arm and straightened out his right leg. Then it spread to the left side, too, and his whole body started to convulse, as if there were electric shocks running through it."

A seizure is a sudden uncontrolled discharge of energy in the central nervous system. *Epilepsy* is the term used for the repeated occurrence of seizures, a disorder that occurs in 1 to 2 percent of the population. Ninety percent of people with epilepsy begin having seizures during childhood or adolescence. Over 70 percent of the seizures in all epileptics can be controlled by anticonvulsant medications.

Seizures may be the result of many different causes, such as metabolic imbalances (sugar, sodium, or calcium that is too high or too low); scars from lacerations or contusions of the brain; infectious diseases (like meningitis); vascular conditions such as strokes; genetic causes; birth trauma; or structural changes such as brain tumors, abscesses, or hematomas. Mr. Lane's seizure was caused by an expanding mass of blood, a hematoma.

During a seizure, the entire body goes into a convulsion with loss of consciousness, and often there is a loss of bowel and bladder control, too. The patient has no memory of the event and feels no pain. Usually there is a period of confusion and/or heavy sleep immediately following the seizure. This period, called postictal state, may last anywhere from a few minutes to a few hours.

The most common serious threat to life during a seizure is spontaneous vomiting followed by aspiration of the stomach contents. Equally threatening is the vomiting induced in the seizure victim by a well-meaning onlooker. The tongue is often bitten during a seizure, and because of the gurgling and gasping that ensues, someone will stick a finger into the victim's mouth to prevent him from choking. This results not only in a bitten finger, but also, and more disastrously, in causing the victim to gag and vomit.

The best thing you can do for a seizure patient is to protect him from hurting himself, by placing a soft object under his head. If you turn the victim on his side, with the head extended back, there will be less chance of aspirating any vomitus. Most seizures last only one or two minutes, and brain damage will not occur unless the seizure lasts over thirty minutes.

After what seemed like an eternity but was actually only a few minutes, Ken's violent shaking and jerking slowed down, and his body relaxed again.

Shortly after the seizure ended, he stopped triggering the Bird machine, no longer capable of making any respiratory effort on his own. His right shoulder, elbow, wrist, and even his fingers were withdrawn into a tight flexion and he was pointing his right leg and foot. This is called "decorticate positioning," indicating a continued progression of the expanding blood clot in Ken Lane's skull. Part of the right side of his brain, the uncus, was being compressed so hard that it was herniating downward toward the spinal cord. His left side was now completely paralyzed.

The left side of the brain supplies nerve fibers to the right side of the body, the right side to the left side of the body. The fibers cross over at or about the level of the upper part of the neck. Thus a person with a compression of the right side of the brain will show symptoms on the left side of the body, and vice versa. The pupil of the eye, however, dilates on the same side as the injury because there is no crossing over of the nerve fibers to the pupil.

I glanced up at the clock. It had been thirty-five minutes since I first told Alice to call Dr. Schepper.

"Alice," I roared, "get Dr. Schepper's answering service on the line. I'll talk to them myself!"

My experience with answering services has taught me how overzealous they can be when trying to shield their doctors from "bothersome" calls. It's one of the things they get paid for. But there are times, and this was one, when I couldn't allow it.

When Alice called out that she had them on the line, I went to her desk. As she handed me the receiver, she backed away from me a little bit.

The tone of my voice was just as grim as I knew the expression on my face must be as I said, "This is Dr. Sword. To whom am I speaking?"

"This is Operator Twenty-nine."

"Okay, Operator Twenty-nine, you listen and listen carefully. This is not your usual afternoon headache call. This is the emergency room at Memorial. We have a man here who has had a serious head injury. He's rapidly turning sour on us, and he's going to die within the hour unless Dr. Schepper operates on him. So you find the good doctor, wherever he is, and you get him down here."

When I hung up the phone, Mark was waiting. "Dr. Sword," he said, "would you believe I drained one and a half quarts of urine from that man's bladder? He's got to be our most grateful patient of the day."

My mood lightened somewhat and I actually managed a smile. Which is how it goes in the emergency room—you veer back and forth, depending on what's happening with the patients under your care. For the sake of my own psyche, I was about to go and see the expression on my "happy" patient's face, when Mr. Lane's X-rays arrived. They showed a long thin fracture line running across the side of his head, exactly where the right middle meningeal artery crosses. Ninety percent of adults who suffer epidural hemorrhages also have associated fractures, while with children it is 50 percent. All seven cervical vertebrae in Mr. Lane's neck were in alignment, so at least he didn't have a broken neck.

As I was studying the X-rays, Alice informed me that Dr. Schepper's office had called, and that he was on his way. I heaved a sigh of relief. My expression must have reassured Alice, because she asked me again if I couldn't please talk to Mrs. Lane.

"All right," I said. "Send her into the doctor's room."

I empathized with the acute anxiety I knew the woman must be feeling. But until a few moments ago, all I could have told her was that her husband desperately needed a neurosurgeon. Now I could at least tell her one was on the way.

She was a sandy-haired woman in her twenties, pale under her freckles. She looked at me with frightened gray eyes.

"How is Ken?"

"Not good," I replied. "The X-rays show a skull fracture on the right side, and he's bleeding rapidly into his brain. Dr. Schepper, our neurosurgeon, should be here any minute. We're getting the operating room set up now."

"He isn't going to die, is he?"

"I don't know, Mrs. Lane."

"Oh, God, can't I be with him?"

I took her to her husband's bedside. When there is nothing left to do but wait, I always wonder if there is some spiritual, noncorporeal level on which people can comfort those they love. I hope so.

When I passed by the admitting desk after leaving Mrs. Lane with her husband, Alice stopped me. "Dr. Sword, I know what you've just gone through has been difficult—but believe me, it could have been worse."

"What do you mean?"

"I mean, I can remember a time when there were *no* doctors available in the emergency room; when patients and their relatives had to wait, sometimes up to an hour, for any physician to arrive. Nurses did what they could, but that was limited by rules and regulations, and by what they knew how to do. You were here for Mr. Lane, and you did a great deal. Think about that, why don't you?"

I stared at her nonplussed, and then I grinned and almost hugged her. "Goddamn, Alice," I said, "if you could bottle those silver linings, you might make a fortune. In fact—"

The sound of a siren outside the doors at the end of the corridor cut off what I was about to say. Moments later, the doors opened with their customary *whoosh* as the paramedics wheeled in a young man with long hair and blood smeared all over his face. Two policemen were following closely.

"What happened?" I asked as they wheeled him to the second bed in the critical care area. Gloria pulled the curtain separating Mrs. Lane and her husband from the half of the room where we would be working on the new arrival.

"The garbage collectors found him lying in back of the Surf Bar," one of the paramedics responded. "They almost backed over him. Nobody even knows how long he was there. The garbage collectors called the police, and the police called us."

"Why didn't you alert us on the biocom?"

"We were just down the street. We figured it would be faster just to 'scoop and run' than to open up the frequency."

"Okay. What's his level of consciousness?"

"No response to verbal commands or shaking, but if you rub his sternum, he'll moan and move his arms and legs."

"How about his pupils?"

"Both slightly dilated. Sluggish reaction to light."

"Well, let's get him undressed and see if he has any other injuries."

The paramedics transferred him from their gurney to ours, and Gloria and Shirley started undressing him.

"He's absolutely filthy," Gloria exclaimed. "Looks like he hasn't had a bath in a year."

Shirley wrinkled her nose. "He smells like stale beer. Year-old stale beer."

"Any ID on him?" I asked.

"Nope. He's been picked clean as a whistle," Shirley answered as she pulled off his pants.

"I wonder how old he is," Gloria murmured.

Shirley shrugged. "Who knows? With his face swollen like an overripe melon and covered with all that dried blood, there's no way of telling. Phew! His socks are almost stuck to his feet."

Looking at his naked body, I judged him to be in his twenties. I didn't see any other injuries, so I said, "Let's look through his hair and see where all that blood came from."

Gloria bent down, then straightened back up quickly, her eyes saucer-wide. "Is that what I think it is?"

I looked where she was staring and felt the hair begin to rise on the back of my neck. The white fragments imbedded in his hair were chips of bone around holes in his skull, and the white stuff obtruding from those holes was his brain. "Get X-ray down here," I said grimly. "And when Dr. Schepper arrives, tell him I need to talk to him. Mark, it isn't going to be easy, but try and shave his head, okay?"

Mark nodded dazedly. "I've never seen anything like this. His brain is actually oozing out of the holes in his skull. He must have been worked over by a claw hammer."

He reached for the razor and started to shave off the hair. I watched in silence until he was almost finished, then asked, "How many holes?"

"I counted twelve. But there are so many cracks and loose pieces of bone lying on top of each other, it's hard to tell where one ends and the next one begins."

I've seen and dealt with a lot of violence, a lot of brutality, but I found it difficult to comprehend how one human being could have done this to another. I've come to believe that people who maim other people should be made to live with their victims, day after day, and nurse them back to health: feed them, wipe their drool off, bathe them, dress them, help them to the toilet, and clean them afterward. Having to go to prison and sit inside some cell block is too easy.

Dr. Schepper stepped in briefly as he was on his way to operate on Mr. Lane. When he saw our latest victim, he shook his head. "Any other weapon, and the man would be dead. But the claw hammer made burr holes, and the burr holes relieved the pressure on his brain and let him live. Start an IV with mannitol and steroids to see if we can get some shrinkage. And give him some antibiotics, too. He's likely to develop meningitis and abscesses. I'll operate on him just as soon as I've finished with Mr. Lane."

Mark and Gloria and Shirley moved into action to carry out his orders, and I stood back and reflected on how nice it was to have two generals on the firing line, instead of one. I wasn't allowed to dwell on that particular reverie very long, however, before Alice's mellifluous voice penetrated my consciousness. "Oh, Dr. Sword . . . we have four patients waiting: a girl bleeding from her ear, a little boy with a lump on his head, a man with something in his eye, and another man with a cut in his scalp."

I went to her desk, glancing up at the clock. It was 1:04 P.M. on a Thursday. "Alice, where do you suppose all these people come from?"

Alice glanced down at her paperwork. "Well, Miss Johnson was working in a bar, and Mr.—"

"It was just a rhetorical question, Alice. I didn't really expect an answer. Where should I begin?"

"Try Miss Johnson on bed four."

Miss Johnson, as it turned out, was a lovely place to begin. She had long black hair, ivory skin, lavender eyes, lips the color of pomegranates. She was still wearing her barmaid's outfit—a low-cut blouse that went way beyond revealing cleavage, and a flared skirt that didn't quite make it to the tops of her thighs. She was wiping tear-wet mascara off her eyes with her right hand when I came around the curtain and holding her left ear with her left hand.

"Hi," I said.

Her eyes brimmed over with tears as she looked at me. "You're not going to believe what happened to me," she said.

"After working here for seven years, I'll believe anything. Try me."

"I'm a waitress at the Green Olive . . . that's why I'm dressed like this." She looked down, then up again. "I don't know why you should have to dress like this in order to serve drinks. Do you?"

I didn't really know how to answer that, and she went on.

"Anyway, some guys at the bar were arguing over the bill. I wasn't paying much attention . . . it goes on all the time. So this one guy reaches down, takes off his leg—can you believe that? I mean, he just reaches down and takes off this wooden leg . . . and throws it at the other guy. The other guy ducked but the wooden leg kept going and landed on the side of my head. And now I can't hear out of my left ear." She started to cry softly.

"Hey," I said, "it'll be okay. Let me have a look. Are you dizzy?"

"I was at first, but I'm not now."

Gloria had arrived and was staring at the young woman sympathetically. I asked her to get me a small metal suction tip so I could clean the debris and blood out of the canal.

Traumatic perforation of the eardrum most commonly occurs when cotton-tipped applicators or bobby pins are pushed into the ear canal too deeply. But a slap to the ear—or a blow from a wooden leg—can also cause a traumatic perforation.

I picked up my otoscope and peered inside, talking as I did so, trying to get Miss Johnson to relax. "I can see a small, irregular tear in the drum itself still oozing some blood. These small tears usually heal of their own accord in a week or so. The drum is actually only thin skin and will repair itself like any other tear in the skin. There's nothing for you to do. Don't irrigate the ear canal with water, or use any ear drops. The loss of hearing is probably caused by blood in the middle ear, which will slowly be absorbed, and your hearing will gradually come back. After I suction out your ear, I'll put some cotton in it to remind you not to put anything else in there. This means no swimming for a while, and baths would be better than showers. I want you to see an ear specialist, an otolaryngologist, in a week to see how the healing process is coming along. So remember," I finished, "put nothing in your ear smaller than your elbow."

I was rewarded with a smile. "Thank you, Doctor."

"All in the line of duty," I said. "Any time you get hit with a wooden leg, you just come to me."

"Onward," I said to Gloria. Almost in cadence, we walked around the curtain to the next bed.

A little boy was sitting on its edge, and his distraught mother was pacing up and down the confined space within the small cubicle. When she saw me come around the curtain, she said, "Oh, Doctor! I'm so afraid Kevin has a tumor. I was combing his hair this morning, and I felt this lump. I *know* it wasn't there yesterday."

The child sat quietly while I began to explore his scalp. It didn't take me long to find the lump and recognize what it was. "It isn't a tumor," I said. "It's a tick, swollen full of blood."

"A *tick?*"

I nodded.

"But how could he have gotten a tick?"

"Probably when he was playing outdoors . . . or with his dog, if you have one."

"Are you sure that's what it is?"

"I'm more sure about this than anything else I've seen today," I said smiling. "Come and see for yourself."

Reluctantly, she drew near and looked where I was pointing.

"See the gray body swollen with blood? Its head is imbedded deeply in the scalp. Ticks have exoskeletons, which means they breathe through their shells. I'm going to put a little mineral oil on its head to make it release its grip. The mineral oil will clog the micropores of its shell, suffocating it and causing it to release its head from Kevin's scalp. Trying to pull it out could leave the head still imbedded in Kevin's scalp and cause an infection later on."

After removing the tick from Kevin's head, I continued on around the next curtain where a bald middle-aged man was sitting on the edge of the bed, his face buried in his hands.

"Hi, I'm Dr. Sword," I said. "What happened to you?"

Without removing his hands from his face, he said, "Shit, Doc, I don't know. I got off working the swing shift, had a beer for breakfast, went to bed. I woke up about six hours later and my eyes were killing me. Feels like there's sand in them."

"Let's have a look. Take your hands away from your eyes so I can see them."

He put his hands down, saying, "The light hurts them."

"Were your eyes okay when you went to bed?"

"Yeah."

I didn't see any foreign material in his eyes, but the whites looked like a road map of the Los Angeles freeway system.

I said, "I'm going to instill a few drops of fluorescein stain and look for corneal scratches" (which will show up bright green under a Wood's lamp, an ultraviolet light).

I put the drops in and a few seconds later, his cornea showed diffuse stippling. "Have you been looking at a welder's arc or using a sun lamp?" I asked him.

"Yes, but that was over eight hours ago."

"Radiation or ultraviolet rays can cause injury to the eye without immediate symptoms," I told him. "What develops is a foreign-body sensation, photophobia or painful sensitivity to light, tears, and pain—all caused by exposure of the free nerve endings on the corneal surface to ultraviolet light. I'll put some drops in your eyes, which will cause the pupil to dilate. It will also reduce your discomfort."

"When will my eyes get better?"

"The outer layer of the cornea will repair itself in twelve to twenty-four hours. We'll give you some patches to wear while you're sleeping, to immobilize the lids and allow healing to take place faster. If your eyes aren't a hundred percent better by tomorrow afternoon, or if they're worse in the morning, you had better see an eye doctor right away."

"Okay, Doc. Thanks."

As I left him, I peered behind the curtain surrounding bed 4. Miss Johnson, alas, was gone. "Where's the fellow with the cut in his scalp?" I asked Gloria.

"Bed three," she said, suppressing a smile.

I walked down the corridor and around the curtain enclosing bed 3. A man I judged to be in his mid-twenties, his sun-bleached hair stained with blood on the crown of his head, was sitting on the edge of the bed staring down at his tennis shoes.

"So," I said, "what zonked you?"

He looked up. "Would you believe a front tooth?"

"It's not quite as colorful as a wooden leg," I said, "but yeah, I'll believe it."

He looked confused.

"Tell me about it," I said.

"Well, I was playing basketball, see, and I gave this guy that was guarding me a head fake. He took the fake, so as I came up he was bending over me, and I hit my head on his mouth. It didn't hurt much. It bled for a little while, but I think the other guy got the worst of it. One of his front teeth was knocked out. Everybody else is still back there looking for it."

I bent down to look at his scalp. "Here. Let me wipe away some of this blood so that—" I straightened up, grinning. "I'll tell you . . . those guys aren't ever going to find that tooth on the basketball court."

"Why not?"

"Because it's imbedded in your scalp."

"*What?*"

I motioned for Gloria to give me a clamp, and then I took hold of the tooth and pulled it out. "Here."

"Jesus, wait till I show the guys." He took the tooth, and stood up as though he was going to leave, as though he'd gotten what he came for.

"Hey, wait a minute," I said. "You have a small cut, about half an inch long. I'll shave an area around it, wash it out with peroxide, and throw in a few stitches."

His expression became glum as he sat back down. "Can you use the dissolvable kind, so I don't have to come back?"

"No. We usually only put dissolvable sutures inside the body, not outside. Most dissolvable sutures are made of something called catgut, which is really sheep gut—and don't ask me why they call it catgut, because I don't know. Catgut sutures lose their strength in five or six days. Another type that has been impregnated with chromatic salts lasts for ten to fourteen days, and the newest type, made of polyglycolic acids, keeps its strength for two or three weeks. This may sound like a long-winded answer to your question, but the point is that dissolvable sutures are made of substances that cause skin reactions, producing swelling, redness, and more scarring. That's why we don't use them on the outside of the body. Nonabsorbable sutures are made of silk, nylon, polyester, or stainless-steel wire. These are inert materials that cause much less of a skin reaction."

He was staring at me with kind of a dazed look. "You always do that?"

"Do what?"

"Answer questions like that?"

"Part of my job," I said.

"Yeah?"

I nodded. "Yeah. Now. I want you to either come back here or go to your family doctor to have your wound checked in two days, and again to have the sutures removed in seven days. You can't swim, but you can wash your hair if you dry it quickly."

I must have sewn up thousands of such lacerations over the past seven years. Most lacerations I see are less than three inches long. Usually I enjoy suturing. I've learned "the trade" by a little reading and lots and lots of practice, and I think I've gotten pretty good at it. Ninety-eight percent of the lacerations I see in the emergency room are such that I feel I can do just as good a job as a plastic surgeon, and I charge a tenth to a third as much money. If a patient finds a scar unacceptable after it has fully healed—and it can take as long as twelve months for this to happen—then at that time a plastic surgeon can be consulted.

Most lacerations should be sutured within twelve hours after they happen, and optimally within the first six hours, which we call "the golden period." This is when an infection is least likely to occur. Lacerations over twelve hours old are often left open to granulate (heal) in slowly "from the bottom up." Sometimes these can be closed secondarily in two to four days.

If there's a problem with bleeding from a laceration, it should always be treated with direct pressure rather than a tourniquet.

If the laceration is in a highly visible place, and the patient or the relatives of the patient ask for a plastic surgeon, then, of course, I'll call one. I never try to talk anybody out of a plastic surgeon, even if I feel I could do just as good a job myself. Many of the people who insist on plastic surgeons are people with unrealistic expectations, and I'd just as soon not be the one to have to deal with them.

Usually, whether or not I call in a specialist depends upon my own assessment of how good a job I can do, and how critical I feel the results are. Children or young adults with facial lacerations are more apt to prompt me to call in a plastic surgeon than, say, a chronic alcoholic who has just fallen on his face for the umpteenth time. I'll also call in a plastic surgeon if I'm extremely busy. I can't, for example, spend a couple of hours sewing up someone's face on a busy Saturday night. But most of the time, it's difficult to get a plastic surgeon to come into the hospital at night. And they definitely won't come unless a patient has verifiable medical insurance. If I need a plastic surgeon at night to work on a Medicaid patient, I'm always told to send that patient to County.

By the time I'd finished up with the basketball player, Ken Lane was coming out of surgery. Dr. Schepper had made an initial burr hole, half an inch in diameter, slightly above and in back of the right ear and just over the fracture line on the right side. This relieved the pressure. The craniotomy was then enlarged to allow for more extensive intervention in order to tie off the bleeding artery. Mr. Lane was lucky. He still has weakness on his left side but he is able to walk with a cane.

As soon as they wheeled Ken Lane out of the operating room, our claw-hammered John Doe was wheeled in. He was there for five hours while Dr. Schepper and the operating team picked the hair and bone out of his brain, after which he spent a month in the intensive care unit—although he would never be fully recovered.

During the hours John Doe spent in surgery, the emergency room quieted down considerably. In fact, the next patient who was admitted struck me as not being an emergency at all. He was a nine-year-old healthy looking boy named Bruce Iverson, whose major problem seemed to be a loquacious, overly concerned mother. After she had gone on interminably about the fact that Bruce's appetite was poor, that he seemed absent-minded, that some days all he wanted to do was sleep, I almost got the impression that she had brought Bruce in to see me because neither of them had had anything better to do that afternoon. I mean, there are days when my own son Tod's appetite is poor, when he's absent-minded, when I think it's going to take a hoist and crane to get him out of bed. Sometimes it signals that he's getting a cold or the flu, sometimes an inner conflict he can't verbalize. I certainly can't picture my wife's taking him to the emergency room because of any of these symptoms.

At the same time, I know mothers often sense things about their children that are difficult for them to put into words. They feel something is wrong, but they don't know what it is. And they're right often enough so that I have learned to listen to them patiently, and probe for information.

"What made you decide to bring Bruce in today?" I asked Mrs. Iverson.

"I don't know. He just doesn't seem right to me. One of his teachers called yesterday and said Bruce's work has fallen off. She said he's been sitting by himself in school, which he's never done before. She asked if anything was the matter at home. I told her about his lack of appetite, how he forgets things, and she suggested I take him to a doctor. Then when I asked Bruce if he'd been having any trouble in school, he said no."

I listened intently, then turned and addressed the boy directly. "Bruce, have you been sick?"

"No."

"Do you hurt anywhere?"

"My head hurts."

"Now that's the first time he's ever mentioned that," his mother said defensively.

"How long has your head been hurting you, Bruce?"

"I don't know."

"Where in your head does it hurt?"

"Over here." He pointed to, and then held, the left side of his head.

Immediately I was concerned. It's unusual for a child to complain specifically of a one-sided headache unless he has seen his parents complain of similar headaches.

"Bruce, have you fallen lately and hit your head, or has someone hit you in the head?"

"No."

"Wait!" Mrs. Iverson said. "About two months ago, he came home from school crying, saying he fell off a swing and hit the left side of his head. There was a goose egg, but I didn't have a car at the time, so I just put some ice on it. When his father got home from work with the car, we were going to take him to the doctor. But the doctor's office was already closed, and David was feeling better. Also, his grandmother was coming for dinner. He said he felt fine the next day, and wanted to go to school, so I thought everything was okay. I never did take him to the doctor. I should have, shouldn't I?"

"Don't start blaming yourself, Mrs. Iverson," I said firmly. "Sometimes these things just don't show up right away."

The history she had given me was quite typical of a subdural blood clot. An epidural blood clot, the kind Ken Lane had, is due to bleeding from an artery; the pressure on the brain increases rapidly, so the symptoms show up immediately. With a subdural clot, the bleeding is from the low-pressure side of the circulation system, the venous side. This slow ooze from a broken vein may delay producing symptoms for months. The clinical picture is far less specific for subdural bleeding than for epidural bleeding.

The examination of the boy revealed very little, which is also typical of subdurals. He was alert and oriented as to person, place, and time. He did not have amnesia. His pupils were okay. He could move his neck and head readily. There was no blood behind the eardrums, and his hearing and eyes were normal. He could move his legs and arms without difficulty. The only thing I noticed was some weakness in his right arm and leg, but this could have been due to the fact that he was left-handed.

"I want to get an X-ray of his skull to see if there are any old fractures," I said after the examination. "However, the X-rays will show only bone, not tissue—which is what we are primarily interested in. So after the X-ray, we'll get an echoencephalogram, a device that uses ultrasonic sound waves to determine the position of the midline of the brain in the skull. It's simple and painless and safe, and all Bruce has to do is lie still. I'm also going to consult with a neurosurgeon to see if there is anything else we should be doing."

The skull X-ray did not show any old or healing fractures. However, the echoencephalogram did show a shift of the brain of about one-half inch to the right, which meant something on the left side was pushing it over. When I talked to Dr. Schepper, he said he wanted a C.A.T. scan, an abbreviation for "computerized axial tomography." In a C.A.T. scan, 28,000 X-ray beams are scanned across an area (in this case, the skull) and deflected on the other side. Using a computer, it is possible to reconstruct a cross-section of the densities in the area scanned, which is displayed on a TV screen and videotaped. The test shows us the exact size and location of a hemorrhage. The patient has to remain still during a C.A.T. scan, which takes about an hour, but the procedure is painless. Radiation from the new-generation C.T. (computerized tomography) scanners equals only two or three chest X-rays. The cost is usually three to six hundred dollars, whereas a skull X-ray costs only about fifty-five dollars.

Bruce was taken to the operating room later that day. A large old clot was found on the right side of his brain, a smaller one on the left. Twenty percent of the time, bleeding occurs on both sides. Since the brain is very soft and the skull very hard, you can think of a blow to the skull almost like a blow to the side of a swimming pool. The blow strikes on one side, but waves of force go across and hit the opposite side, too. So when force or pressure on one side of the skull is transmitted to the opposite side, bleeding occurs on both sides.

Shirley, always inquisitive, always curious, always wanting to learn, asked me later if a lumbar puncture, or spinal tap, would have been helpful in diagnosing what was wrong with Bruce. I told her that a spinal tap should never be done if there's any possibility of intracranial pressure. If the pressure inside the head is high and you pull fluid out from below, the brain is pushed downward. This results in herniation and puts pressure on the medulla, which controls breathing.

In fact, today, with the ready availability of the echoencephalogram and the C.A.T. scan, there's seldom any reason to do a spinal tap unless you're looking for bacteria or a virus, as in meningitis.

I know many people are afraid of spinal taps. They picture the needle damaging the spinal cord. In actuality, this just doesn't happen. When I do a spinal tap, I position the patient in a curled-up position on his or her side, which opens the spaces between the lumbar vertebrae. I clean the skin just down from the top of the hip bone and numb the area with some lidocaine. The needle I use, three and one-half inches long, is inserted between the fifth and fourth vertebrae or between the fourth and third, but no higher. At this level, the spinal cord is divided into many strands, like a horse's tail—hence the name *cauda equina*. When the needle is passed between them, the strands of nerves are just pushed aside. In my mind, I aim the needle at the umbilicus, and I go in until I feel a "pop." This occurs when I penetrate the tough dura matter that covers the brain and continues on down covering the spinal cord. A teaspoon or two of the spinal fluid is then removed and sent to the lab for various tests. Normally, the spinal fluid is crystal clear, like water. But if meningitis or some other infection is present, we see white cells or pus in the fluid. We keep the patients lying down for a few hours after the tap to avoid what has become known as a "postspinal headache." This headache is probably due to the loss of spinal fluid. Lying down will minimize the headache's severity until the body has had a chance to replace the lost fluid, which it does within a few hours.

As I was waiting for Bruce Iverson's results, I remembered a three-year-old boy who had been brought in by his father the week before. The man said his son had fallen against the corner of a coffee table. The boy wasn't even crying, just smiling and looking around, enjoying all the attention. He had a cut about three-eighths of an inch long right in the middle of his forehead. It had stopped bleeding, and, in fact, hardly seemed worth sewing up. But I dutifully put on a pair of sterile gloves and explored the cut with my little finger. The wound was deeper than it looked, and as I probed, the boy started to cry.

"Can you tell me more about how this happened?" I asked the father.

"We were just about to get him ready for bed. He was playing with his older brother when he fell against the table and hit his head."

"Was he knocked out? Did he lose consciousness?"

"No, he got up right away. It was bleeding a lot at first, but we put some ice and a cloth over it, and it stopped. I wasn't even going to bring him down here, but my wife insisted."

"Well, it feels a little deeper than I thought," I said. "I'd like to get a skull X-ray before I sew it up."

The father frowned. "Do you really think that's necessary? I mean, it was only a little fall. He wasn't even knocked out. And I'm the one who has to pay for the X-ray."

"I know," I said. "But I try to handle each patient the way I would if he or she were a member of my own family. If this were my son, I'd want an X-ray."

He sighed. "All right. Go ahead."

I understood his position. Sometimes it seems as though 99 percent of all skull X-rays turn out to be negative for fractures, and they are expensive. Skull films cost about $55. When this is added to the $22 emergency room fee, $5 for a tetanus shot, $15 for a sterile suture instrument tray, and my $40 professional fee for suturing, it comes to $137.

Nevertheless, there are three axioms for an EM physician to follow: Always do what you feel is best for the patient—not just what is convenient, or costs the least, or is expedient; if it hurts, X-ray it; and never try to save money in the ER, since the only one who will thank you is the patient's lawyer.

I always try to back up my subjective clinical judgment with objective evidence. And in cases where my judgment tells me there is only a 1 percent chance a child has a fracture, when I order an X-ray I'm probably doing it to "cover my ass" in case I have to go to court later. Certainly I considered this child's X-ray in that category. But when the film came back, not only did he have a skull fracture, but an area of bone the size of a silver dollar was depressed against the brain. He needed immediate surgery. One incident like that justifies, in my mind, a thousand cover-my-ass X-rays.

The day had been a long one, and the dinner hour was approaching. Since I'd already had a claw-hammered skull, a wooden-leg-clobbered ear, and a tooth-imbedded scalp, I figured I might just get through the rest of that Thursday without incident.

I was wrong. While I was picturing myself walking into my house, peering inside the pots on the stove to see what was for dinner, City Rescue called to say they were bringing in a victim with a gunshot wound to the head. They were coming in Code 3, with an ETA of three minutes.

I started barking out the orders again, as I'd already done several times that day: "Get Respiratory Therapy down here right away. Have X-ray standing by with their portable. Get the lab on the phone, have them stand by for possible type and crossmatch of blood. Get the IV tray set up, normal saline. Get a bottle of mannitol ready, too."

Bullet wounds to the head are extremely dangerous for several reasons. Not only do the bullets cause bleeding and serious damage to the brain tissue, but there's a shock wave of destructive force that surrounds the bullet. When it hits the skull, the bullet will break apart and drive in contaminants of hair, cloth, and spicules of bone, producing a shotgun effect. The spicules of bone and fragments of metal can spread all over and become the source of epileptic seizures in the victim in years to come—assuming he even recovers from the initial injury.

Mark had positioned himself near the door to watch for the paramedics. "Here they are!" he announced.

The opaque sliding glass doors opened, and the paramedics wheeled in a Mr. Weaver, a forty-eight-year-old Caucasian male. Following closely were Mr. Weaver's wife, his two children, and several policemen.

Mr. Weaver was shouting, "Let me die! Let me die!"

Mr. Weaver's family followed his gurney right into the critical care area. His children were crying, his wife moaning. The policemen came in, too, talking to each other. The noise level was deafening.

"Get his wife and kids out of here!" I shouted at the police, the clear implication being that I wanted them to leave, too.

Then I turned to the paramedics. "What happened?"

"The way we got the story, he took a twenty-two-caliber pistol, placed it behind his right ear, and pulled the trigger. He did it at the dinner table right in front of his wife and kids."

"Lord."

"Ever since we picked him up, he's been yelling, 'I want to die, let me die!'"

"What IV do you have running on him?"

"Normal saline. We got it going on the way in."

When I examined Mr. Weaver, he seemed remarkably intact for a man who had just shot himself in the head. He was alert and conscious, his pupils reacted normally to light, he could move all his extremities, and his reflexes were normal. The bullet's entrance wound was just behind his right ear, but I couldn't see an exit wound. I could tell the pistol had been held very close to his skull, since the entrance wound was a small hole about the size of a pencil and there was a charred area about the size of a half dollar surrounding it. What I couldn't understand was how he could still be alert, and sitting up and looking around.

I ordered a portable X-ray so I could see the location of the bullet, then went to talk to his wife. She said he was depressed about his job, their deepening financial crisis, and the fact that life seemed to be "passing him by."

When the X-rays came back, they were really puzzling. The bullet was lodged between the bone and skin on the left side, even though he had shot himself on the right side. I decided the X-ray film must be mislabeled as to left and right. The X-ray showed the bullet lying so close to the skin that I thought I should be able to feel it.

I went to Mr. Weaver's bedside, and felt carefully under the charred area. Nothing. So I felt behind the other ear, and there it was.

Mark had been following my examination closely. "How did it get over there?" he asked.

"It's the damnedest thing," I said. "Apparently the bullet went in on the right side at such an angle behind the ear that it traveled around the back of his head. It must have traveled the whole way between the scalp and the skull, lodging on the left side of his head just behind the left ear at almost the identical place it went in on the opposite side."

"You're sure it didn't just go straight across?"

"If it had," I said, "he wouldn't have been yelling when they brought him in. It's right here, just beneath the scalp. I think I can remove it. I'll just shave his scalp about one inch square around it, make a small incision with a scalpel, take it out, and sew the wound back up."

Everyone on the staff was as amazed as Mark and I were. After I took out the bullet, I trimmed the burned, dead tissue from the entrance wound, leaving it open with sterile gauze over it for skin grafting later. I gave Mr. Weaver a tetanus shot, started him on some antibiotics, and went to offer the bullet to the police.

They declined it. They had no further interest in the case.

So I offered it to Mr. Weaver. "How about it, Mr. Weaver? Do you want it as a souvenir?"

"Go to hell, Doc. Just go to hell!"

Hell? Not me. I was going home to dinner. I was going to sit down at the table with my wife and kids and put the Ken Lanes and the John Does and the Mr. Weavers of the world out of my mind.

Until tomorrow.

9

Out, Up, or Down

A CURIOUS PATTERN exists among the drug-overdose victims I see in the emergency room, one that seems to break down into male and female. Most men shoot heroin, or play drug roulette with LSD or PCP. If a woman overdoses on one of these, it's usually because she's "doing" drugs with a man, or because a man has gotten her hooked. The drugs a woman overdoses on—on her own—are usually the "safe" prescription drugs some doctor has prescribed to help her cope or help her sleep. She turns them, instead, into a one-way ticket to oblivion. Almost all the female overdose victims I see are attempted suicides. The male overdose victims are, I think, seekers of the grail; "last frontiersmen" attempting to wrest, through drugs, an identity-defining adventure that their twentieth-century urban existence denies them.

Seven out of ten drug-overdose victims are women, and two to six times as many women as men suffer from depression. Perhaps women are so vulnerable to depression because emotional attachments are more important to them than they are to men, and in our society they are often denied these emotional attachments.

I'm convinced it was the erosion of her personal relationships that pushed Clara Chapman over the edge. Clara, a woman in her early thirties, was brought in last week by two young paramedics —neither of whom thought she was going to make it.

"She's real deep," one of them said as they wheeled the stretcher in.

"Too late," the other one said. "I know we were too late on this one."

A glance at the woman told me that she was indeed in deep trouble, and I yelled down the corridor to Gloria to call Respiratory Therapy and get them down here *stat!*

Then I turned back to the paramedics. "How did you find her?"

The one who had spoken first answered me. "Her landlord got suspicious when he didn't see her leave for work. He checked her parking stall and saw that her car was still there, but she didn't answer the door or her phone, so he called the police. They forced their way in and found her lying on the floor unconscious."

"She lives alone, then?"

"Apparently. Landlord says she got divorced a year or so ago. She has three kids, but they're living with the father."

"Well, let's get her up on bed one. Does her landlord happen to know what she took, or when she might have taken it?"

The other paramedic fumbled in his pocket and withdrew an empty prescription bottle and a folded piece of paper and held them out to me. "These were on the table next to her bed," he said.

As they transferred the woman up onto the bed in the critical care area, I read the label on the prescription bottle: "Clara Chapman . . . Seconal . . . 100 mgm . . . take one at bedtime as needed . . . 50 dispensed . . . Dr. Jones."

Dr. Jones. Dr. *Who* Jones, I wondered. Whenever I'm confronted with a patient who has taken an overdose of sleeping pills, I wish I could haul the doctors who prescribe them down to the emergency room to see their "sleepless" patients on the verge of death; then maybe they'd start paying more attention to the cause of the sleeplessness instead of just treating the symptom.

The prescription was dated ten days ago. I started to count it out. If she'd taken the pills as directed, she should have forty left. Even if she'd doubled the prescription dosage, she'd still have thirty left. Only she didn't have any left. I had to figure she'd taken between 3.5 and 4.5 grams . . . a fatal dose.

Gloria came hurrying into the critical care area to tell me she'd called Respiratory Therapy and a technician was on the way. Then she looked down at Clara and asked, "What did she take?"

I handed her the prescription bottle and the note. She glanced at the bottle. "What does the note say?"

I shrugged. "Read it."

She unfolded the piece of paper slowly and began to read:

> Dear Mike:
> I'm sorry, but I can't take it any longer. I've suffered enough. I'm tired of living. When I met you, I thought things would change. I never loved a person like I loved you. I take your picture wherever I go. I know both of us have our own life to follow, but I'm tired of mine. Mike, I'm sorry. Take good care of the boys.
>   Clara

Gloria had started reading the note in her normal tone of voice. When she finished she was almost whispering, and her eyes were bright.

You never know when it's going to hit you, this sudden caring about someone. You work in the emergency room so long—and Gloria had been here longer than I—and you figure you've seen it all, felt it all; nothing can get to you anymore—until suddenly it nails you to the wall. Like my choking up when I had to tell Mrs. Gootee her husband might not make it. Like Gloria now, with this woman. Is it because chords are struck in our own psyche? Had Mrs. Gootee somehow reminded me of my own mother when my father was dying? Did this woman remind Gloria of someone, or some aspect of herself?

Most people who overdose on sleeping pills aren't as far gone as Clara when they reach the emergency room. In fact, some people never intend to commit suicide at all: they only want it to look like they tried. I've encountered several women who took a suicidal number of pills just before their husbands or lovers were due to arrive home. And I've also seen some arrive dead, or closer to dying than they ever intended to be, because their husbands or lovers were delayed at work, or caught in traffic jams on the way home.

Clara, of course, hadn't expected anybody to rescue her. Clara had definitely given up on knights on white chargers.

"Let's get her hooked up to the oxygen tubes," I said briskly. "And take her robe off so I can watch her breathing more closely. Gloria, help me sit her up for a minute so I can check her back. I once had what I thought was a suicide who turned out to be a stab wound."

I didn't find any bruises or wounds, so I laid her back down. When I examined her pupils, I found them dilated but still reacting sluggishly to light. Her deep tendon reflexes—ankle, knee, and elbow—were all absent when I checked them with my rubber hammer. The gag reflex, which keeps food out of the trachea, was also absent.

When I checked her pain threshold by running my knuckles against her sternum and then sticking a pin into her index fingers and the soles of her feet, she didn't respond. She was slipping away from us fast.

Greg Adams, the respiration therapist, came around the curtains into the critical care area. Greg has a round, rosy-cheeked cherubic face, and I swear he looked to me like one of Santa's elves at that moment. Greg and I had worked together a few months ago on a saxophonist who had gone into respiratory failure after smoking one too many Shermans (marijuana cigarettes laced with PCP). The guy kept surging in and out of consciousness and each time he was conscious would look up at me and say, "Hey, Dad, what's comin' down?" Since that day, Greg always greeted me with, "Hey, Dad, what's comin' down?"

This time he got as far as "Hey, Dad—" before he stopped. It was clear to him as it was to me what was "comin' down."

"Give me a number eight endotracheal tube," I said, "and then get the Bird set up."

Greg moved silently and efficiently to assist me.

As I explained before, when I do a tracheal intubation I pass an eleven-inch tube directly into the trachea. Open at both ends, the tube contains an adaptor at the upper end that can be attached to a mechanical breathing device, such as a Bird. When the cuff located near the end is sealed, it allows positive-pressure ventilation and keeps the airway from sucking in foreign material, such as vomitus, from the stomach.

I wanted her hooked up to the Bird for fifteen minutes, and then I wanted to get a set of blood gasses, which would tell us how well we were ventilating her.

After I had the tube in place with the cuff inflated, I told Greg to get a chest X-ray to check the position of the tube; I then asked Gloria to check her blood pressure.

"It's one hundred over seventy, with a thready pulse of sixty."

"Start an IV of D_5W, and put in a Foley catheter so we can check her urine output."

Shirley had come around the curtain moments ago. There were now four of us concerting our efforts to save this woman who wanted so badly to die.

"Shirley, have the lab come down here and draw some blood."

She nodded. "What tests do you want?"

At times like this, I always have to remind myself to take a methodical, judicial approach, not let myself jump to any conclusions. While the evidence certainly indicated that Clara had taken Seconal, I didn't know this to be unequivocally true. So whatever tests I ordered would have to not only prove that she had taken Seconal, but also rule out other possibilities as causes of her coma.

Assuming she had taken the Seconal, I would need a barb (barbiturate) level to see how much had gotten into her bloodstream; a drug screen and a blood-alcohol test to see if she'd taken anything else, or washed down her pills with booze; a blood sugar to rule out hypoglycemia or diabetes; a complete blood count to rule out the possibility of any overwhelming infection; a hemoglobin to show up any significant blood loss; a blood urea nitrogen which, in uremia or kidney failure, would be elevated; and finally, electrolytes: sodium, potassium, chloride, bicarbonate, and calcium. If all of the latter were normal, the tests would have ruled out metabolic and more obscure causes of coma.

As I was rattling off the names of all the tests I wanted, I noticed that Greg's cherubic brow was furrowed with concern.

"What is it?" I asked him.

"She isn't triggering the Bird at all anymore," he said. "The machine is doing all her breathing for her."

I glanced at the clock. In five more minutes we could get a blood-gas study.

Barbiturates such as Seconal, depressants, and tranquilizing drugs—including heroin—all act similarly. They all depress the central nervous system, especially the respiratory center in the medulla. If the patient stops breathing, cardiac arrest will occur within a few minutes. The pivot around which all management therapy revolves is the support of respiration by providing breathing via a machine. Once this is done, the liver can usually metabolize the drug, or the kidneys can eliminate it.

At that point I had taken every defensive precaution I could on behalf of the patient in coma. Now it was time to take the offensive. I had no way of knowing when she had taken the pills, but I wanted to remove as much of the Seconal that hadn't been absorbed into her system as possible. That would entail what lay people call "pumping out her stomach."

Actually, there is no pump. What we do is put a size-36 French lavage tube in the nose or mouth and down into the stomach. This tube is about half an inch in diameter, the size of the little finger. Anything smaller than that tends to get plugged up with food fragments, or even the pills themselves. In fact, sometimes a number of capsules will stick together and form a large mass which, if left in the stomach, would take days to dissolve. After we get the tube into the stomach, we pour half a pint of water down the tube and immediately draw it back out. We repeat this, using a minimum of four to five quarts of water, and we keep going until the return fluid is clear.

If Clara had been conscious I would have given her ipecac to induce vomiting, which is what we always use when a drug-overdose or accidental-poisoning victim is seizure-free and conscious (unless the person has swallowed a strong alkali or acid or petroleum distillate, which of itself has probably caused the person to retch; if not, in those cases we give milk). Ipecac is a caramel-colored, cloyingly sweet liquid. The recommended dosage is two tablespoons, followed by a lot of water—most of which the patient will vomit right back up. Sometimes I tell paramedics to give ipecac on the spot, then bring the patient in. Vomiting will empty a stomach more thoroughly than lavaging or "pumping." But if a poison or overdose victim has been given ipecac and hasn't vomited by the time they reach the hospital, I'll put the old tube down and siphon out the stomach.

I told Gloria to initiate the procedure, and the first thing she flushed back were some red fragments. These were the Seconal capsules. Seconal has the street name "reds."

Angry parents or relatives of patients who have overdosed on drugs will sometimes ask me to use the stomach pump as a form of punishment. Needless to say, I don't honor such requests. Most poison and drug-overdose victims have been taught enough of a lesson by the havoc wreaked on their bodies. By the time they reach us, if they're still conscious they'll do anything we tell them to do—including taking ipecac, or accepting stomach lavage.

When Gloria succeeded in getting a clear return on the lavage, I told her to make a slurry of activated charcoal and magnesium sulfate and put it down the hose. The charcoal would bind up any of the Seconal that hadn't been washed out, and prevent it from being absorbed into Clara's body. (Unfortunately charcoal will not bind with all drugs. It doesn't work well, for example, with cyanide, acids, alkaloids, or alcohol.) The magnesium sulfate would act as a cathartic to reduce the transit time of the drug in the intestine, thereby also decreasing its absorption. Magnesium sulfate with the charcoal also acts as an indicator in the stool. When a black stool appears, it's unlikely that any more of the drug will be absorbed.

While Gloria was mixing the slurry, I went to have a look at Clara's lab tests and chest X-ray. Her barb level confirmed, as I had been 99 percent certain it would, that she had taken a large dose of Seconal. Alice had called the pharmacy that had filled the Seconal prescription and discovered that the prescribing doctor worked with a medical group that specialized in welfare patients (a situation discussed further in the last chapter). Doctors whose patient load consists primarily of welfare patients often refer all their crisis cases to hospital emergency rooms and are "not available" when we want to discuss a patient with them. Consequently,

Alice had gone ahead, contacted our on-call medical backup doctor, and had obtained his permission to admit Clara into the hospital. Clara's blood sugar was all right, her kidneys were in good shape, and her CBC didn't show anything unusual. Her blood pressure had risen to 110 over 70 after we started the stomach lavage. When I looked at her chest X-ray on the view box, it showed the endotracheal tube in a good position and her lung fields clear, so things were definitely looking up.

I had the feeling, though, that if Clara had been conscious through everything we'd done to keep her alive, she would have resisted us.

As Jane Linton did.

Before I saw Jane Linton I heard her cursing and shouting in the waiting room, and between her rantings I could hear Alice calling out, "Dr. Sword, could you please come!"

I motioned to Mark to grab a wheelchair, and we headed up the corridor; but before we even reached the door, an overweight, balding, middle-aged man came through half holding up a blowsy, drunken woman. Her blouse was completely unbuttoned, her eyelids drooped, and her knees kept buckling under her.

"You got to help her, Doc," the man was saying. "She took a whole bunch of pills."

I motioned Mark toward them. "Get her into a wheelchair," I told him.

"Don't touch me!" she screamed.

"Do something, Doc," the man moaned.

Both of them reeked like a distillery. I don't have a lot of tolerance for obnoxious drunks, and sometimes I have to work hard just to remain civil to them. So while Mark literally wrestled the woman into the wheelchair, it was in a highly controlled and icy tone of voice that I asked the man, "What did she take?"

"Some kind of nerve pills, I think."

"Do you know the name?"

"No."

"Did you bring the empty bottle?"

"No."

"How long ago did she take them?"

"Maybe thirty minutes, maybe more; I'm not sure."

"How many did she take?"

"I don't know. She . . . uh . . . she's had a lot to drink tonight, too."

Clearly the man didn't know anything that was going to be helpful. "You go on back out into the waiting room now," I told him.

"I'd rather stay with her."

I shook my head. "Sorry."

As he started reluctantly to leave, the woman yelled, "Frank! Don't go!"

He turned around again and said belligerently, "I'm staying."

"I have to get those pills out of her stomach," I countered firmly. "After I've done that, I'll call you."

Scowling, muttering under his breath, he finally went back to the waiting room.

By then the woman was sitting slumped in the wheelchair like a sack of potatoes. I went to ask her the same questions I'd asked the man: What had she taken? How many? How long ago? She stubbornly turned her head away, refusing to answer. I wasn't in a mood to play games. I rubbed my knuckle briskly on her mid-sternum to get her attention and succeeded.

"That hurts!"

"Believe it or not, I'm trying to help you," I said.

"I just wanna go home."

"Not until I get the poison out of your system."

"What do you care what's inside me? I want to die. Just let me die."

"The second you came through that door, lady, you became my responsibility. You're not going to die in my emergency room."

She started to sob. "Just leave me alone."

Both time and my patience were running out. Mark, anticipating me, had brought the ipecac. I held it under her nose. "You'll drink this medicine right now, or I'm going to put a tube down your nose and pump your stomach out."

Her self-pity turned back into anger. She slapped the ipecac out of my hand and started to try to get up. "I'm going home!"

She couldn't stand up, of course, let alone take a step toward the door. And damned if I was going to watch her slide down into a coma. "Mark," I said grimly, "help me wheel her over to bed four and we'll tie her down."

I don't know where she found the strength to fight as she did while we were tying her legs to the foot of the bed with two-inch leather straps. Gloria had come running to help, and the woman managed to scratch her in the face and kick Mark in the stomach, but finally we succeeded in tying her down.

I put some lubricant on a nasogastric tube, held her hair back tightly to prevent her from shaking her head, and inserted the tube. As we washed out her stomach, a lot of undigested yellow pills came back that I assumed were Valium. Once the washings were clear, I put a charcoal and magnesium slurry down the tube before I pulled it out. By then she'd calmed down considerably. I washed up and went out to the waiting room to talk to her husband. He was sitting slumped on the vinyl-covered couch, watching television with dull eyes. He too had calmed down considerably.

"Mr. Linton?"

He didn't respond.

"Mr. Linton?" I said louder.

He looked up. "Huh?"

"Your wife needs—"

He interrupted me. "My name is Reyes and she's not my wife. We live together, but she's not my wife."

Damn. I'd wanted him to sign for her and initiate a seventy-two-hour hold designating her as a danger to herself. But since he wasn't her husband, he couldn't do that. "Well, does your . . . Does she have any insurance? Does she work?"

He shook his head. "She can't seem to hold no regular job."

"Does she have a private doctor? Where did she get those pills she swallowed?"

"Stole 'em," he said. "She cleans people's houses once in a while. She stole 'em."

"Well, look," I said. "The law requires a nurse to be with all suicide attempts for twenty-four hours to make sure they don't jump out a window or do anything else to injure themselves. Your friend needs to spend the rest of the night in a hospital and be evaluated by a psychiatrist in the morning. Since she doesn't have any doctor or any insurance, the best thing I can do is transfer her to County."

He stood up. "No!" he said. "She ain't going to that place. If she has to go there again, she'll kill herself for sure. Why can't you be her doctor? Or get some other doctor to be her doctor?"

"My practice is limited to the emergency room," I told him. "If her condition were critical or unstable, I could assign her to one of our on-call doctors. But I can't force any doctor to accept a patient who isn't critical or unstable. Since she isn't employed and doesn't carry insurance, any doctor I talk to will tell me to transfer her to County."

He grimaced. "It always comes down to money, doesn't it?"

I stared glumly at the man, not knowing what to do. You don't learn a damn thing in medical school that will prepare you for situations like this. If I let her walk out of the hospital right now and she injured herself, I could be held responsible. If, on the other hand, *I* initiated and signed for a seventy-two-hour hold, keeping her against her will, I could be charged with assault. A commonsense approach is what I usually look for—some calm, cool, collected way to try to defuse the situation.

"Listen," I said, "what we really want to determine here is whether she's going to slide into a coma or not. The next few hours should let us know. We've pumped her stomach and given her charcoal. I think she's going to be all right; what she needs is a good night's rest and somebody to watch her in case she tries to get out of bed, or vomits. If a person in a decreased state of consciousness vomits while lying on their back, they're in danger of inspirating the vomit into their lungs, and you have to roll them on their side before that happens. So how about you? Would you be willing to sit with her?"

"If it means keeping her out of County, hell, yes."

"Good," I said. "Come with me."

As I led him back to the woman's bed, I reflected that at least it was a variation on the usual theme of "out, up, or down." Usually we act as a triage in the emergency room. We see patients in the order of the criticalness of their needs, stabilize them, and then send them *out* the door to their homes or to County Hospital;

admit them *up* into this hospital; or send them *down* to the morgue. With Jane Linton, we were simply going to wait.

As it turned out, she fully regained consciousness several hours later and wanted to leave. After reexamining her, I was convinced that what she needed (in the short term) was simply more time to sleep it off. Since I believed her to be out of immediate medical danger, I wasn't going to sign the seventy-two-hour hold form. She, of course, refused to sign herself into a mental center to get psychiatric help, which was what she needed in the long term. So before she left, I had her sign an "against medical advice" (AMA) form which stated that she was leaving the hospital against my advice, and that the hospital and myself were absolved of any responsibility for her.

Let me hasten to add that the AMA form is a fairly worthless piece of paper. Any lawyer could come along and say, in effect, "How can you have someone sign a document when they are under the influence of drugs?" On the other hand, the same lawyer could also argue that keeping someone against their will was an infringement of their rights. So I really can't win. The AMA form is just another piece of paper with which I try to CMA . . . having learned long ago that "covering my ass," or trying to, is an inherent part of my existence in the emergency room.

Some large metropolitan hospital emergency rooms have a "holding ward" where patients like Jane Linton can be kept for observation for twelve to twenty-four hours. There is no such ward in this hospital, and normally I wouldn't tie up a bed for several hours. If Mr. Reyes hadn't volunteered to sit with her, I would have had no choice but to send her to County. But since I did have a volunteer attendant, I figured I could bend a little. If there's one thing an EM physician has to be, it's flexible.

This wasn't the first time, of course, that I'd wished this hospital had a holding ward; I always do when I have patients on bad trips from hallucinogens. So many of them are in their teens—the prime age for a "rite of passage," a "last frontiersman" adventure. After they recover (if they even do), they tell me that they don't understand what happened; that all of their other trips were good ones. But I only see the bad trips.

The cases I really hate are the ones where parents drag their son or daughter into the emergency room and try to get me to "prove" their child has been taking drugs. I'm a doctor, not a policeman. The only medical way to do this is to run a drug screen on a blood sample. Taking blood from someone who is resisting you is extremely difficult, and I won't take blood from a teenager unless I have his or her consent. Assuming I do get a blood sample, it takes two or three days to get the results back. The drug screen itself costs up to two hundred dollars, and usually the procedure is not covered by insurance. Moreover, most laboratories are not equipped to detect many of the street drugs, including pot, LSD, and PCP. If parents think their children are heavily into drugs, they should sit down and talk to them, or go to a counselor who specializes in such problems. An emergency room can't solve a drug problem; it can only try to deal with the bad trips.

Lysergic acid diethylamide (LSD) and phencyclidine (PCP, also called "angel dust" or "rocket fuel") are responsible for most of the bad trips I see. I've heard of hallucinogens being concocted from mushrooms, mescaline, morning-glory seeds, and banana peels ("mellow yellow"), but I've never treated anyone who has taken one of these. I did once see a couple of kids who mixed peanut butter with water and injected it into their veins.

Hallucinogenic drugs aren't addictive. If a person suddenly stops taking hallucinogens, there are no withdrawal symptoms. They pose no problems with regard to respiratory depression as do barbiturates, tranquilizers, and heroin. There is, however, the danger of a "flashback," a replay of a bad trip. Often a patient will suffer one of these days or even weeks after the initial episode—even though he or she hasn't taken any additional amounts of the drug. And thus far psychiatrists and psychologists are not able to predict the individuals for whom these drugs are potentially dangerous.

Paranoia, panic, and fear are the reactions attendant on an overdose of LSD. LSD hasn't been produced in the United States for a couple of years, so any of it obtainable today must come from the black market. Black-market drugs, of course, aren't standardized. LSD is such a potent drug that 3.5 millionths of an ounce is the usual dosage. But with the tremendous variation in contents of the LSD sold on the street, no one knows how much the drug is cut, or what actually constitutes a dose. LSD users say they take the drug so they can "hear" colors and "see" sounds. But these same visual and auditory hallucinations bring on the anxiety attacks that lead the user into confusion, panic, and ultimately end in a bad trip. In the emergency room we try not to physically restrain LSD overdose victims. If they're violent and pose a threat to themselves or others, I will inject Thorazine or Valium intramuscularly. But generally we simply try to talk them down, reassuring them that they are safe. In most cases the symptoms wear off in a few hours, although occasionally they will last for days.

Agitation, flushing, sweating, vomiting, muscle quivering, muscle rigidity, and sliding into a coma are the possible reactions attendant on an overdose of PCP. These are the reactions we can readily cope with in the emergency room. There are a few others, though, that give us a hell of a time. Insensitivity to pain is one. PCP can anesthetize those who use it. I've seen some PCP users with every bone in both hands broken, because they pounded their fists repeatedly against concrete walls without feeling a thing. Superhuman strength is another. A PCP user can break the two-inch leather straps we use as restraints as easily as if they were made of paper.

Jane Linton—drunk, overdosed on Valium, belligerent, and refusing help—wasn't a whole lot of fun, but compared to someone overdosed on LSD or PCP, compared to a gentleman I chanced to meet named, aptly, Leroy Brown, she was a piece of cake.

Leroy Brown was a wild-eyed, muscular teenager brought forcibly into my emergency room by seven of his friends. While six of them fought to hold him down, the seventh separated himself from the struggling mass of bodies to address me.

"You the doc?" he inquired.

I glanced around for Mark, wondering where my karate champ was when I needed him, before I finally (and glumly) said, "Yeah. I'm the doc. What's going on?"

"Old Leroy here has taken some dust. We tried to talk to him nice—but he thinks he's a bird. All he wants to do is get up on a roof and try to fly."

"Well, you tell your friends to see if they can get him up onto a bed in a treatment room," I said.

To their credit, Leroy's friends did their best. But they could only partially hold him. During the ensuing struggle gurneys were sent flying in all directions, and patients and staff alike were yelling and falling over each other to get out of the way. One man who had come in to have his recently sutured head wound checked fell over a wheelchair as he tried to get up, twisted his ankle, and went hopping out the door with his head bandage flapping loosely, running for his life.

Old Leroy was kicking, screaming, cursing, shouting that he wanted to fly, and altogether getting the best of his seven friends.

"Leroy!" I shouted. "I am a doctor. You are in a hospital. Calm down!"

My words bounced off him like tennis balls off a concrete wall. Clearly there was no point in trying to talk to him.

Mark had come running by then (along with Gloria and Shirley) to see what all the commotion was about. I said to Gloria, "Give him a hundred milligrams of Thorazine IM, and see if that settles him down a little."

Gloria looked from Leroy and his friends back to me and blanched a little, but went ahead and got the Thorazine ready. When Leroy—held down as much as he could be held down by his seven friends—saw Gloria coming at him with the syringe and needle, he managed to get one leg loose and kick Gloria in the stomach, knocking the needle to the floor. Shirley dove in to pick it up and got kicked in the chest by Leroy's other foot for her trouble.

Gloria stamped her foot. "That does it. I'm calling the police," she announced. And she left to do just that.

Leroy's friends hadn't liked hearing her say that, but they were just as trapped as the rest of us. If they let go of Leroy, he'd start swinging on *them* now. What they had was a tiger by the tail.

Most policemen have a very protective attitude toward female nurses. They figure male doctors can take care of themselves (which we can . . . usually). But nurses need, and deserve, protecting. It couldn't have been three minutes after Gloria's exit that ten of the biggest boys in blue came pouring into the corridor outside the treatment room.

I knew if I told them to restrain Leroy, one of them would manage to "choke him out" with a hammerlock behind his neck, cutting off all blood to his head until he passed out. Prisoners in custody have been known to have their necks broken and die from such grips. Consequently, I wasn't overly fond of hammerlocks being used in my emergency room. And I doubted if Leroy's friends would stand by peaceably while the police manhandled their buddy.

The situation was taking a rapid plunge from bad to worse. The police were glaring at Leroy and his friends, and Leroy's friends were glaring back at the police. In the ten to fifteen feet that separated the two groups, the aura of hostility was almost visible.

I don't normally have a Superman complex. But I was still holding the syringe and needle I'd picked up, and for some reason I couldn't have explained then and haven't been able to figure out to this day, I stepped into the no-man's land between those two hostile groups and said, "Wait!"

If jaws dropping could be heard, I would have been listening to a veritable chorus.

"I'll give him the Thorazine myself."

Before the police had time to respond, I turned my back on them and said to Leroy's friends, "Listen, you guys, all you have to do is hold him still long enough so I can give him a shot. You can do that, can't you? I mean, there's only one of him, and seven of you."

I think they were just too dumbfounded to object. Inevitably, as I approached him with the syringe and needle, Leroy, who had been surprisingly quiet for several moments, started going crazy again. "Turn him over!" I shouted to his friends. Somehow they did. I don't even know for sure where I stuck him, but within ten minutes he was sleeping like a baby.

Was I a hero?

I was not.

Leroy's friends were angry at me for allowing the police to be called. The police were angry at me for not letting them "take care of" Leroy. The nurses were angry at me for not having taken a more active role in the beginning—if I could do it after the police got there, why couldn't I have done it before? And if Leroy had been awake instead of asleep, he would have been mad as hell at me, too. It was the old can't-win-for-losing syndrome.

Chronic drug users, as a rule, aren't prone to being grateful. Not even when you save their lives.

The heroin victim, for example, whom I wrote about in the preface had to be strapped down when he started to "pink up" and regain consciousness, because it looked as if he might get violent, might pull out his endotracheal tube and injure his vocal cords. The end of his story is that when we finally took out the tube through which we'd been doing his breathing for him he said, "Get these fucking straps off my arms, you bastards."

I managed to ignore that and ask him, "Do you remember what happened to you?"

"Sure. I was with some friends and passed out."

"Do you remember shooting up some smack?"

"Hey, I don't touch that stuff, man."

"So what are those tracks up and down your arms? Been practicing your needlework?"

"Fuck you, man. I used to use the stuff. But not anymore. Now let me get the shit out of here."

It's a familiar story. A bunch of users, two or three or more, get together to shoot it up, sharing spoons, syringes, needles. There's no telling why this guy had taken too much, though it may have been because there was a new shipment of heroin on the market. We often get a rash of overdoses then, because the new stuff isn't cut as much with fillers. Sometimes we'll get two or three overdoses a night for several nights running, but it will drop off as suddenly as it began.

The last thing this guy remembered was being in a house or garage and shooting it up with some other people. He had no memory of being in a critical condition, and he just wouldn't believe he'd been snatched from death's jaw. Fortunately, his friends had known enough to bring him to us. They were afraid of the police and didn't want to get involved, so they'd just dumped him out of the car next to our emergency room door.

Sometimes friends will carry an overdose victim in, saying they "found" him—after they have made certain he has no drugs on him for the police to find. When I turn around to ask them more questions, they've gone.

I could have asked the police to book this guy, but I knew what they would have said:

"*You didn't find any drugs on him, did you?*"

"*No.*"

"*Then he's all yours, Doc.*"

"*What if I sign a seventy-two-hour hold on him?*"

"*He'd be out on the streets at the end of the seventy-two hours faster than you could finish writing your report. Save your time for the people who need and appreciate your efforts.*"

"Are you going to let me out of your fucking booby hatch or aren't you?" the addict was demanding.

Sometimes it's hard not to take the verbal abuse personally. Once in a while my emotions get the better of me and I react. I'll look at one of these young addicts and say something like, "Who or what gives you the right to destroy your mind, destroy your body . . ."

I didn't this time. Instead I said, "Will you consent to go to the county hospital for drug rehabilitation treatment?"

He looked at me incredulously. "Are you kidding?" Then he started to laugh.

I let him use a phone to call a friend to come pick him up. There wasn't any point in doing anything else.

When I told him to sign an AMA form before he left, he said, "Fuck you, man. I ain't signing nothing!"

I knew if he was dropped at our door tomorrow or the next day or the next, not breathing, within moments of dying, we'd all labor just as hard to save him as we had this day.

Saving lives is our job. It goes, as they say, with the turf. We do it the best we can.

10

No Humans Involved

ONE ASPECT of emergency medicine particularly sets it apart from other medical specialties, and that is the frequency with which we must work with the police. They are present so often in the emergency room—especially on Saturday nights and holidays—that I sometimes think they work there, just as I do. They accompany victims of small and large catastrophes. Often it is left to them to bring in those whom society has abandoned: the ill, injured, or dying derelicts found in alleyways, in dingy "single-room occupancy" hotel rooms, in ancient and rundown apartment buildings. The police bring in the child-abuse victims—*and* their parents. They bring in members of street gangs who have knifed or shot each other, and the innocent bystanders who have been knifed or shot by street-gang kids. As a matter of routine procedure, they bring in drunks for blood-alcohol testing in order to ascertain just how intoxicated they are. And they bring in suspects they want medically examined or cleared before they book them into jail.

If a suspect on the way to jail tells the police he's a diabetic, or an asthmatic, or has a bleeding ulcer, that suspect has a ticket to see me for a prebooking exam. If he tells the police he has a heart condition or epilepsy and needs his pills, then he will be brought to me. If a suspect has been "roughed up" during his arrest and the police believe he's going to yell "police brutality" after he's been booked, they bring him first to me so the actual extent of his injuries can be verified prior to booking. They will also do this with a prisoner who has been known to bang his own head against the bars of his cell and then claim police brutality. Or if a suspect is arrested with pills in his possession and claims the pills made him do whatever unlawful thing he did, he is brought in to the emergency room.

Occasionally I'm also called on to give postbooking exams. If a suspect who is already in jail complains that he's going into the DTs, is suffering withdrawal from drugs, or is in severe pain for any reason the police will—if the suspect convinces them that the pain or injury is real—bring him to the ER for an examination. They much prefer a prebooking medical exam to a postbooking one because they have to fill out papers to get the prisoner out of jail for the latter, and two police officers must escort the prisoner to the hospital and wait while the examination is taking place.

Three courses are open to me when I give either prebooking or postbooking exams: If I judge a suspect to be in critical condition, I can say that person must remain with me until I can render him stable; I can send a suspect who isn't in critical condition but needs medical treatment to the special jail ward at County Hospital; or, if a prisoner is neither ill nor injured and I feel he needs no medical attention, I can tell the police it's safe to take that person (back) into jail.

Most suspects would prefer being booked into the jail ward at County to being booked into regular jails because the living conditions there are better.

Most of the police, however, would prefer to have me say "okay to book" so they can take their prisoners to the local jail. To drive a prisoner downtown and book him into County takes several hours of a policeman's time. And if that policeman is due to go off duty soon, he doesn't want to put in the extra hours. For that reason, I sometimes get caught in the middle. Suspects for vagrancy or intoxication have been brought in for prebooking exams; I have discovered possible cases of hepatitis or tuberculosis that would necessitate the police transporting the suspects to County ... and presto! The vagrancy and/or intoxication charges were dropped. I've even heard the police say, when I thought there might be a fracture and I ordered X-rays to find out, "If he has a fracture, we'll let him go. But if he doesn't, we'll book him."

When cases are borderline the police may try to pressure me a bit by saying things like, "Doc, he doesn't need to go to County . . . he'll bail out in the next few hours anyway." Or, "We know this guy, Doc. He's always pulling this stuff."

However, the final decision is mine, and if I feel a suspect's condition warrants hospitalization, I won't hesitate to order the transfer to County.

The personalities and temperaments of the police I work with are just as diverse as those of the rest of the population. Sometimes I get along with them and sometimes I don't. I think many of our disagreements stem from the fact that they are policemen and I am a doctor. They try to enforce the law; I try to save lives. They see one side of life; I see another.

As I've said elsewhere, on occasion I get angry at some of my patients. I don't like to be spat at or threatened or insulted. Yet I never forget my patients' humanness—and the fact that they are in my care. Some of the police I work with not only do not acknowledge the humanness of certain of their prisoners, but in some cases they deny it. There is a phrase they use when describing certain cases they are involved in: "N.H.I."—no humans involved. In gang wars, for example, between ghetto minorities, they will say, "N.H.I."

The police see the violence, and I see the victims.

The police expose themselves to the violence, while I mend, or try to mend, those to whom violence has been done.

I guess it's not surprising that we have divergent points of view about some of the people we both have to deal with. We saw Olu Apia, for example, through different eyes. . . .

Olu Apia was a nineteen-year-old Samoan boy who had been shot six times at close range with a .38 Special while holding up a liquor store. The police had radioed that they were bringing him in on a "scoop and run." When a victim is found by police or paramedics so close to the hospital that it would take less time to bring him to the hospital than it would to treat him on the scene, they bring the patient directly to the emergency room. This is called a "Scoop and Run."

By the time the police cars came screaming up to the ambulance entrance, I had Inhalation Therapy, X-ray, and the lab standing by, and Shirley was preparing several bottles of normal saline. Four officers, one on each arm and leg, carried Olu in as if he were a sack of fertilizer. His head, limp and bobbing up and down, almost hit the floor as they threw him onto the gurney. His color was ashen gray; he was unconscious and scarcely breathing.

Ignoring the police and everyone except my patient, I moved into action, telling the inhalation therapist to get an endotracheal tube down his throat and start bag breathing him, telling Mark to check his blood pressure and hook him up to the monitor, telling Gloria to start an IV in his left arm, and Shirley to start one in his right. Then I began to work on establishing a CVP (central venous pressure) line so we could start pouring fluids into him. I palpated the place where the external jugular vein crossed the strap muscles on the side of his neck, two to three inches above his clavicle. I guided a number 14 intracath needle under the strap muscles for about two and a half inches until I saw a surge of dark blood filling the syringe—which meant I was into the vein. Then I threaded a catheter eighteen inches through the needle until it reached the right side of the heart, removed the needle, and left the catheter in place.

The lab technician arrived and I told her to get Olu's blood typed and crossmatched, then get ten units back to us as fast as she could.

By that time Gloria and Shirley had their IV lines going in his left and right arms and Mark, getting a thready pulse of 140 but no pressure, had put a Foley catheter up into his bladder.

I listened through a stethoscope and couldn't hear any breath sounds on the right side. I started to look for the bullet holes and found two in the right chest, one in the right hand, and one in the right shoulder. I knew I was going to have to put a chest tube in him, so I told the X-ray technician to do a chest plate and Shirley to get the tray ready. While they were doing that, I started to look for the last two bullet holes. Rolling him over, I saw number five between his shoulder blades and number six in the back of his right shoulder. I was afraid number five might have gotten his spinal cord, because I'd already noticed he had a slight erection, which is a sign of traumatic rupture of the spinal cord. When I rolled him back, I checked his reflexes. He had none below the waist.

"How's his breathing?" I asked the inhalation therapist.

"I'm still breathing for him. But he tries to take a breath on his own once in a while."

"How much fluid have you gotten in him?" I asked Shirley.

"Two and a half liters and still pouring in."

"Keep it going," I said, "and after that third bottle is finished, hang on a bottle of plasma."

"Pressure's up to seventy over zero," Scott informed me. "Pulse still at one forty."

The chest plate was ready by then. It showed his right lung completely collapsed and full of blood. If I didn't put a chest tube in soon, the blood would push over and compress his left lung. Taking a scalpel, I made an incision just below the seventh rib under his right arm. By blunt dissection, I quickly pushed a clamp over the top of the seventh rib and through the pleura. Once the tube was inserted the blood poured out and I was able to drain off three liters rapidly.

Finally I stood back and asked myself if I was doing everything I possibly could. An endotracheal tube was in place, so we were controlling his respirations and airway; fluid was pouring into him from three IVs; blood was on its way; a Foley catheter was in place to measure his urinary output; the chest tube was draining the blood out of his chest; X-rays had been taken that showed the location of the bullets.

I told the X-ray technician to get another chest plate, to show the location of the chest tube, then sent Shirley to get hold of the on-call thoracic surgeon. Finally, I told Gloria to put a nasogastric tube down into his stomach and hook it up to low suction.

"That'll be six tubes and lines in him," she said as she worked.

I nodded. Sometimes I think there is an inverse relationship between the number of tubes and lines we put into a patient and that patient's chances for survival: the greater the number of tubes and lines we have to put in, the less chance he has of making it.

"How's his pressure now, Mark?"

"Eighty-five over zero."

Shirley came back to tell me she had the thoracic surgeon on the phone and I went to talk to him. When I described Olu's wounds, he agreed to take him into surgery within the hour.

On my way back down the corridor, one of the policemen who had brought Olu in stopped me. "Is he going to live?"

"If he does, he'll probably never walk again," I replied.

"Yeah. Well, he got what he deserved."

I was curious to know what kind of crime deserved six bullets at close range. "What did he do?"

"He goes into this liquor store, see, and draws a gun on the owner. He forces the owner into a walk-in freezer and goes for the cash register. The owner of the liquor store has been held up twice before, so he keeps a thirty-eight Special in the freezer. The Samoan can't get the cash drawer open, so he gets the owner out of the freezer to unlock it for him. And when the guy begins to gather up the money, the owner pulls out the gun and lets him have it."

"Six times," I said drily.

"Sure, six times. You figure it's the third time this guy's been held up, he's entitled."

The lab technician arrived with the ten units of blood I'd ordered, so I didn't have time to continue my discussion with the police officer.

Olu Apia, as it turned out, lived. He entered the courtroom in a wheelchair, paralyzed from the waist down, and was sentenced for armed robbery.

Samoans are physically beautiful people, and Olu Apia was typical: tall, well built, brown skinned, good looking. I don't know why he tried to steal. Whatever the reason was, did it render him less than human? I can't accept that, though I think I can guess what the police would say: "You face him while he's holding a gun on you, and then tell me how human he is."

Facing death every day on the streets gets to them, I know. So they react. And one way they alleviate the pressure is by developing their repertoire of insults. Sometimes they'll bring in a suspect they've managed to devastate with insults. Homosexuals are their favorite prey, and they call them "peanut-butter packers," "poop shooters," "Hershey Bar–expressway users," and "shit-chute drillers." Minorities, drunks, and drug addicts are referred to as "PPPs" (piss-poor protoplasms), "SHPSs" (subhuman pieces of shit), and "FUBARs" (fucked-up beyond all recognition).

When police bring suspects whom they've angered to the point where they're out of control into the emergency room, I'll try to calm them down, telling them I'm a doctor and not associated with the police. I don't always succeed in getting through to them—they'll see me in my hospital coat as just one more uniformed authority figure who is going to denigrate them, and they'll refuse to let me examine them, refuse treatment.

Eddie McCoy, for instance.

I think even on one of his good days Eddie would have been just about the meanest-looking teenage tough I've ever seen, and the day I saw him definitely wasn't one of his good days. He was one of those tall, strapping kids whose muscles seem to ripple under their skin. When two officers brought him in, his face and neck were covered with blood. The oldest officer, a veteran whose time on the force was mapped in the lines in his face and the grim expression in his eyes, said, "We caught this one impersonating a human. Thought you might want to look at the little cut on his head."

Blood from Eddie's scalp wound had streamed down onto his face and neck. Because scalp lacerations bleed so profusely, they usually look much worse than they are. The bleeding can be stopped by simply applying pressure directly on the wound for twenty to thirty minutes. Eddie's wound, I could see, was no longer bleeding.

"So what happened?" I asked Eddie.

Before Eddie could answer, the younger of the two officers said, "One of his friends popped him."

"The Pigs hit me!" Eddie countered. "The fucking Pigs."

"Well, look," I said; "right now it doesn't matter who hit you. You have a cut that probably could use a few stitches, so let me have a look at it."

As I started to approach him, he growled, "You ain't touching me. Stay away."

I stopped in my tracks. I knew he meant it.

"You have to understand, Doc," the veteran policeman said. "He wants to show off his blood to his friends, and if you clean him up, there won't be anything to show off but that little cut."

The younger officer chimed in, "Hell, he may even be able to convince his lawyer we beat him up."

Then it was Eddie's turn. "You bet I will, Pig!"

"He's okay for booking, right?" the veteran officer said.

I hesitated briefly. Clearly it was going to take Eddie hours to calm down enough so I could get near him. And equally clearly he was going to survive without the two or three stitches I could have put in his scalp.

I told the two officers to go ahead and book him.

After you've seen a hundred Eddies you begin to accept the fact that you're never going to find out who did what to whom. So you concentrate on finding out what happened, how it happened. Even if a prisoner has a broken arm, I've learned to ask what happened and how, not who did it. And after you've seen a hundred Eddies, you almost forget how caring the police can be when they do regard the prisoners in their custody as fellow human beings.

Frank Mason, for example. Frank Mason was an emaciated old man who looked as if he would blow away in a medium-sized gust of wind. When the police brought him in, I wondered what he could possibly be guilty of. He scarcely looked strong enough to tie his shoes, let alone commit a crime.

One of the policemen sat down beside Frank on the chairs lining the walls of the corridor, and the other officer motioned me to one side.

"He says he needs his heart pills, Doc."

"Is he having chest pain?"

"Shit, I don't know. He didn't say he was hurting. All he said was he needed his heart pills. You know what we have to book him for?"

I shook my head.

"He was caught shoplifting a dollar sixty-nine worth of hamburger. We wouldn't have brought him in—hell, *I* would have paid for the damn hamburger—but the store manager is a real bastard and filed a complaint against him."

"Well, I'll talk to him and see what kind of pills he needs."

The other police officer was sitting on the old man's right, so I sat down beside him on the left. I could see he had been crying. Before I could even speak, he focused his rheumy old eyes on me and said, "I'm sorry I took the food. The checkout girls know me; they pretend not to see what I do. I only take a few things . . . meat's so expensive these days. My wife's an invalid, she needs me at home. What is she going to do without me?"

I didn't know how to answer that. The officer sitting on his right told him, "Don't worry, Frank. You'll be out within an hour after we get you to the police station."

The old man didn't seem to hear him.

"Are you having chest pain, or shortness of breath?" I asked him.

He didn't seem to hear me either. "You see, I mix the meat up with some dog food so my wife won't know. Meat goes a long way when I do that. You won't tell her, will you?"

"We won't tell her," I said. Then I looked across him and spoke to the officer. "He doesn't seem to be in any pain. If he's going to be released in an hour, there's no use my giving him any medication. I'd just be guessing what to give him, and I'm not sure he even knows what he takes."

The officer sighed. "We'll go ahead and take him in, then."

I watched them leave, the two police officers with the frail old man between them. I'd seen those two in action a few times, and I knew they could be as tough as any of their brethren on the force. Yet they were being as tender with Frank Mason as they would be with their father.

It's curious and mysterious what reactions other human beings evoke in us. Two other officers had brought in an old woman the week before, Flora Dorrity. The younger officer wouldn't look at me and kept blowing his nose. I knew it wasn't the smog, and I also knew he didn't have a cold. They'd found

Flora in a filthy hovel on Congress Street. Someone had called the precinct, given her address, said it sounded as if someone were being choked to death.

The two officers told me they'd found hundreds of baby-food cans and jars all over the inside of that hovel.

When I went to examine Flora, I asked her how old she was. She said sixty-five, but she looked ninety-five. Her neck felt as hard as wood on the left side, and on the inside of her mouth there was a pinkish cauliflowerlike mass growing out from beneath her tongue. When I saw it, I felt a shiver go up and down my spine. The growth was cancer, and so far advanced that it was literally choking her to death. She'd been surviving on baby food. Now I doubted she could even get that down.

She told me she'd never seen a doctor, that she thought her "problem" would go away by itself.

What do you do when you have to deal with something like that? I don't know. Sometimes I find myself taking sidelong glances at other cultures and wondering—if the Chinese, the Indians can honor their elderly, why can't we? Sometimes I even end up preaching a little. I found myself giving my staff an angry sermon that afternoon on the fact that people need to be educated to take care of themselves. They'd all seen Flora. They knew why I was preaching. So they nodded their heads and agreed with everything I said. Actually, everything I said was true.

Years ago, the government of this country decided that many grave medical problems developed because people couldn't see a doctor, and all it had to do to obliterate a lot of sickness was to make sure everyone had access to a doctor. Well, within a five-square-mile radius of the hovel Flora Dorrity lived in, there were probably twenty-five doctors and two hospitals. So access to doctors wasn't the answer. Educating people so they'd know when to see one has to be the answer—educating them so that when something goes terribly wrong with their lives, they know enough to seek help.

The Flora Dorritys of the world aren't the only ones who move me to preach sermons. Victims of child abuse also move me to step up on a pulpit.

One form of child abuse—an indirect, often unintentional,

but nevertheless a deadly form—is exposing children to poisonous substances. Accidental poisoning is a leading cause of death in young children. Somehow, some way, the general public must be made aware of the number of accidental poisonings that occur annually in this country—more than 1 million, 10 percent of all admissions to urban general hospitals. Kids reaching for bottles of pills that look like candy. Kids getting hold of beverage bottles filled with stuff that looks like soda pop. Can you believe that twenty thousand hospitalizations (90 percent of whom are children under five) occur each year because people fill carbonated beverage bottles with oil or kerosene and leave them within reach of small children? Two teaspoons of many common household fluids can be fatal. Many doctors are hesitant to induce vomiting in these cases, because it increases the chances of the patient's aspirating the toxic stuff into the lungs and contracting a severe form of pneumonia. On the other hand, leaving the poison in the stomach can lead to coma and death. A real "damned if you do, damned if you don't" situation.

That's one form of what I consider child abuse that rankles. The other, of course, is the blatant form.

The last child-abuse victim I had was a three-week-old infant brought to me off a transcontinental jetliner. A stewardess had noticed a young mother trying to force solid food into her baby's mouth. When she offered to prepare some warm milk, the mother sullenly refused the offer. The stewardess watched the woman closely during the rest of the flight and believed she saw the mother being abusive to the infant. She told the pilot, who radioed ahead for help.

When the plane landed, two policemen were waiting to talk to the mother. Seeing them, the woman literally threw the child at them and ran. It took both police officers as well as three airport security guards to subdue her. (One thing police hate to do is subdue a female. They say no matter how strong she is or how violently she resists them, inevitably they're accused of police brutality.) As it turned out, this particular woman was wanted in her home city for armed robbery.

I never saw the mother, but her baby was brought in for an

examination before being placed in a foster home. The infant girl was dirty, malnourished, and had a severe diaper rash.

I considered this child lucky: She'd been rescued from an abusive parent before any severe or lasting harm had been done to her.

In this country, 100,000 children a year are known victims of child abuse—not only physical abuse, but also drug abuse, sexual abuse, nutritional neglect, medical neglect. These are the children somebody notices, tries to help. God only knows how many more are out there that nobody sees—or if they do see, they pretend not to.

Five percent of these children die, victims of a single severe physical attack. Thirty-five percent suffer brain damage and associated mental retardation as a result of repeated attacks.

Those of us who work in hospital settings are tempted, of course, to blame the parents of these children. But that's almost like blaming a sick oak tree for producing unhealthy acorns. So often the parents who abuse their children were abused by their own parents. You'd be inclined to think that since they themselves had suffered, they'd be the last ones to mete out pain and suffering. Instead, a convoluted pattern has been set in motion, trapping them in a destructive cycle.

There is an organization called Parents Anonymous that can help them if they know how to ask for help. Just as the members of Alcoholics Anonymous are alcoholics who have helped each other stop drinking, the members of Parents Anonymous help each other stop abusing their children.

But not all child abusers are themselves victims of child abuse. Sometimes—and no one really yet understands this phenomenon—a scapegoat pattern is set in motion in a particular family and one child is singled out for abuse by the rest of the family members. Usually the one singled out has some aberrant personality trait or behavior syndrome—hyperactivity, for instance—upon which the attacks are focused.

And sometimes child abuse within a family unit is triggered by economic and/or emotional crises: Poverty, a death in the family, even a divorce can become so unendurable for an adult that finally he or she lashes out at the children.

All fifty states now have laws requiring physicians to report cases of suspected child abuse. It isn't neccessary that a doctor be able to prove the suspicions. Any physician making such a report is assumed to be acting in good faith and is immune from civil or criminal liability. But when a physician doesn't report a case of suspected child abuse, he becomes liable to both criminal and civil actions. A number of negligent-action suits have actually been brought against doctors who failed to report cases of child abuse.

Emergency medicine physicians are likely to see more child-abuse cases than do other doctors. Consequently I and all the other emergency physicians I know have learned to maintain a high index of suspicion. We look for certain points in an ill or injured child's history:

- Has the child been a patient in several hospitals in the recent past?
- Did the injury for which the child was brought to the hospital occur several days earlier?
- Is the nature of the injury consistent with its alleged cause?
- Are the parents' reactions appropriate to the severity of the injury?
- Do inconsistencies in what the child says and what the parents say appear after repeated questioning?
- Does the child show signs of neglect—such as malnutrition or poor skin hygiene?
- Does the child have bruises in various stages of healing?
- Is the child either irritable or overly subdued?
- Do the parents have a history of alcoholism or drug addiction?

After it has been established that a case of child abuse does in fact exist, we join with other professionals in trying to convince the parents that they must accept help. Until a decade ago, people believed that taking a child away from abusive parents was the best solution. Now most experts agree that both the child and society as a whole are better served by teaching the parents to alter their behavior patterns, by showing them ways to change their attitudes toward themselves as well as toward their children.

It has been found that 10 to 15 percent of parents who abuse their children can't be taught these things, can't change, can't find their way out of the negative pattern their lives have taken. But 85 to 90 percent do change, do learn ways to accept themselves and their children. So educating people to become aware of their options seems to be the best answer in this case, as in so many others.

But not everyone is willing to learn or to listen. Beverly Larkin, for example. Beverly Larkin was a twenty-nine-year-old woman the police brought in for a prebooking exam before they put her in jail for shoplifting.

I don't know what I was expecting when I walked down the corridor and around the curtain of the bed where she was. I guess I had a mental image that didn't let me think a shoplifter could be attractive. Attractive . . . Beverly Larkin was gorgeous. Huge eyes. A cloud of dark hair. Cranberry lips. But she also had a breast oozing pus.

While I examined her, she told me that after having three kids within a two-and-a-half-year span, her once beautiful breasts lost all their tone. So she'd decided to have an implant done. She found the name of a plastic surgeon in the yellow pages of her phone book. The man (I can't seem to bring myself to call him a doctor) put disks in her breasts that were so large she felt they made her look like a freak. So she went back to him to have the large disks exchanged for smaller ones. These were all right in size, but after a time the disk in her right breast started moving up until that breast was several inches higher than the left one, and she couldn't raise her arm. She went back for corrective surgery, after which she thought everything was going to be fine. The size was right, the position was right. Then her right breast started to become tender, so she again went to see the man. He assured her that her condition was normal for so soon after surgery. He removed her sutures—and two days later the incision under her right breast started to separate and ooze pus.

When I saw her, her left breast was beautifully shaped,

though it felt like putty. Her right breast was badly misshapen, and protruding from underneath the breast mound was the smooth blueish lip of a plastic disk. Angry-looking inflamed skin surrounded it, and pus was oozing down her belly.

I told Beverly that the disk would have to be removed until the infection cleared up—that once an area with a foreign body becomes infected, you almost always have to remove the foreign body in order to clear up the infection. After the infection cleared up she could have another disk inserted—but I didn't think it would be a good idea to go back to the same plastic surgeon who'd fouled her up three times already.

She shrugged. "I paid him," she said. "He owes me."

What could I say to that? I told the police she needed to be booked into County for medical treatment, and they took her away. Some people are slow learners.

Drunks are slow learners. Drunks are never my favorite people to work on—but that may be because I'm overexposed to the species (I understand that doctors who tend athletes seek out fat, indolent people in their off-duty hours). The police bring in at least one drunk for blood-alcohol testing on every shift I work. On weekends and holidays, the average is two to three per shift.

I won't draw blood from any conscious person—sober or drunk—unless they sign a consent form first. Most people who are suspected of being intoxicated while driving will end up signing, because if they refuse to consent to any of the required trio of tests (which includes a breath test, a urine test, and a blood test for alcohol), they lose their license for six months.

All I do is draw the blood and turn it over to the police for analysis. If the blood concentration of alcohol is above 0.10 percent, a person is considered legally intoxicated. The body can burn off about one ounce of alcohol per hour. So two or three beers or one mixed drink consumed in less than an hour will usually result in a blood concentration of alcohol above the legal limit. If a person who weighs 150 pounds spreads his liquor consumption so that he has three drinks over a three-hour period, he should maintain a passable level of sobriety.

Occasionally, and I always hate it when it happens, I'll have to not only draw blood but also attest to someone's sobriety.

Flight personnel, for instance, are required to refrain from consuming alcoholic beverages for twelve hours prior to a flight.

Just last month I had to examine a flight attendant who had been taken off her scheduled flight because her pilot believed she was intoxicated. Her supervisor brought her in. The woman stubbornly denied being intoxicated, but she couldn't do the heel-to-toe test while walking a straight line, nor could she touch her nose with her finger on the first, second, or even third try. I had no choice but to attest that in my opinion she was under the influence of alcohol.

She lost her job. Two weeks later she showed up with a lawyer wanting to know exactly what tests I had done. She *had* signed a consent for the blood sample I drew, and her recorded blood level of 179 milligrams percent (.179) substantiated my opinion that she was intoxicated. Nevertheless, I expect to have to go to court on this one. It may be months or even years from now, but I'll probably have to go.

Her case wasn't as distressing as the last so-called drunk I had (who turned out not to be a drunk at all). His name was Bill Adams. The police had picked him up for speeding through a red light. He'd told them he'd had a few beers, so they were bringing him in for a blood-alcohol test when he started talking about his chest hurting.

The police, figuring he was trying to wriggle out of the drunk-driving charge, hadn't paid too much attention to what he was saying about his chest.

But I didn't like the way he was hunching his shoulders. After a few years in the emergency room, you learn to distinguish fairly accurately between "real" pain and "fake" pain. This guy's pain seemed real to me.

I told him to take his shirt off and sit up on bed 4, then asked him when the pain had started.

"It's more like pressure than pain," he said. "Like a three hundred-pound canary sitting on my chest. It started when I saw the red lights of the police car behind me. I knew I was going too fast, but when I saw the traffic light change I knew it was too late to stop, so I just gunned it."

"Have you ever had pressure or pain like this before?"

"Once in a while I'll get pressure in my chest if I work too hard. But it goes away if I sit down and rest for a few minutes. It's never been this bad."

His pressure was 140 over 90, his pulse strong and regular, and his skin color good. But I still didn't like the way he was hunching his shoulders. I told Gloria to get him on the monitor and asked Shirley to start an IV and give him some oxygen.

As Gloria was pasting on the last of the four electrodes and Shirley was getting the oxygen hose around his nose, he suddenly stopped talking, became stiff, and gasped deeply.

"Look at the monitor!" Gloria exclaimed. "He looks as if he's in V-fib" (ventricular fibrillation).

I glanced at the monitor, and then at the leads. The leads were all in place. The man's heart was beating about six hundred times per minute, which was essentially no effective beats at all. I had about four minutes to get his heart beating effectively again or we were going to lose him.

I asked Gloria for the defibrillator paddles and she thrust them at me. As I said, "Turn the current up to 400 watts," I noticed there wasn't any conduction paste on the paddles. "You forgot the paste," I snapped.

She was looking all over the countertop. "I can't find it," she moaned.

I didn't have time to worry about the damn paste. I placed the paddles—one under his right collar bone, one under his left nipple—and pressed the button. He jumped, arching his back and neck. No change on the monitor. I pressed again. Once more he jumped and arched up, and then he blinked and opened his eyes.

He was in a normal sinus rhythm, with his heart beating strongly and regularly.

He looked down at his chest. There were two red, round second-degree burns on his chest where I had put the paddles. "Jesus, Doc," he said, "what'd you do?"

My forehead was beaded with sweat. I fumbled for an answer. But before I could speak, he said, "Whatever it was did the trick. Pressure's gone. Want me to do the heel-toe walk now?"

I swear these bizarre cases go in cycles. The night after I saw Bill Adams was the night I saw Jimmy Rollins, whom I will not ever forget.

Alice told me a young man with a laceration of his lower lip was waiting to see me on bed 5. When I went around the curtain, I saw a young guy sitting on the edge of the bed. He looked nervous to me, a little jumpy, but I figured it was because his lip hurt.

"What happened?" I asked him.

"I cut myself," he snapped.

"I can see that. How did you do it?"

"I ran into a clothesline. Look, what difference does it make? Just sew it up. You'll get paid."

Clearly I wasn't going to find out how it had happened, so I concentrated on the wound. It was about three-quarters of an inch long, just under his lower lip. His teeth seemed intact. I told him I was going to numb his lip with Novocain and then sew it up. I figured a few sutures on the outside and some on the inside would take care of it. But while I was injecting him, I found a half-inch cut on the inside of the lip and another one below the teeth, just at the base of the gums. Then I noticed how all the time he'd been sitting there he'd been bleeding and swallowing the blood.

I tried to suture the cut at the base of the gums first, but I couldn't get the lower lip out of the way so I could see clearly. I called Gloria and told her to put on a pair of gloves, then hold the lower lip down so I could see better.

She noticed the bleeding right away. "Where is it all coming from?" she asked.

"Apparently from this cut I'm trying to sew up," I said, starting to show that fine edge of irritation I always feel when I'm getting into trouble.

"Do you want me to use the suction?" she asked. "Maybe you could see better."

I nodded.

For twenty solid minutes I tried suturing the inside of Jimmy's mouth. The position was awkward. The light was hot. I couldn't seem to get a good bite into the tissue with my suture needle. I tried different needle sizes, different thicknesses of catgut, but they kept tearing the fragile mucous-membrane tissue at the base of the gums. I even tried putting a suture through the bone—and only succeeded in breaking off the needle point and having frantically to retrieve it.

The bleeding continued.

I wasn't paying attention to the time, or to anything but the war between Jimmy's gums and me. It was one of those moments in my career when I was looking at the tree and missing the forest.

Finally Gloria cleared her throat and said, "Doctor Sword . . . maybe you'd better look at the suction trap."

When I glanced at it, I couldn't believe what I saw: There was nearly a pint of blood in it. I looked back at Jimmy. At Jimmy . . . not just his mouth. He was sweating.

"Gloria," I said tensely, "deglove, and take his pressure."

She did so quickly. "It's one hundred over seventy. The pulse is one twenty and thready."

I felt cold perspiration begin to trickle down my back, drop by drop. This young man was bleeding to death before my very eyes and I couldn't seem to stop it.

I yelled for Mark, then told Gloria to start an IV of normal saline, and after she'd done that, to have the lab come over *stat* to type and crossmatch him for four units.

When Mark came running, I told him to get the oral surgeon who was on call on the phone. "Don't take any flak from the answering service," I said. "Tell them it's urgent."

Then I put a pressure dressing in Jimmy's mouth, but he continued to bleed bright red blood around it.

Mark returned moments later to tell me he had Dr. Booker on the phone. I left Gloria and Mark with Jimmy and went to talk to the oral surgeon. I knew that I sounded like a scared intern as I explained the problem. Hell, I felt like a scared intern.

"Well, Dr. Sword," he said soothingly, "you've got the IV in and running, and you have blood for transfusing being prepared. Keep his blood pressure up, pack some sterile fine-mesh gauze tightly into his mouth and under his lip, and relax. I'll be right down."

As I hung up the phone, the police arrived. They were looking for a suspect who had tried to rob a billiard parlor and had gotten a pool stick jammed in his face for his trouble. None other than Jimmy Rollins. I told them they'd have to wait a while for Jimmy, that he couldn't go anywhere just yet.

Dr. Booker arrived a few minutes later. He wasn't a particularly awesome-looking man, but to me he looked at least ten feet tall.

With the help of some special retractors from the operating room, we found the problem. The pool cue had gone through the lower lip and had broken the thin bony plate that holds the teeth in place. It had also severed the two arteries that supply blood to the teeth. Had I known this initially, I'd never have tried to suture him up myself.

Dr. Booker got the bleeding under control. We gave Jimmy two units of blood and let the police take him to County Hospital. The police couldn't understand, of course, why I'd been so concerned about somebody being hit in the mouth with a pool stick. "Jeez, Doc," one of them said. "You'd think he was dying or something."

I gave him a tired grin. "Yeah," I said. "You would."

11

Rape – the Invisible Crime

IT WAS ONE OF THOSE NIGHTS that have a kind of suspended echo to them. You know the feeling . . . as if you're waiting for the other shoe to drop.

I don't mean to imply that it was a quiet night, because it wasn't. On one bed we had Mrs. Ellis, age fifty-three, recently arrived from St. Louis for a visit with her newborn granddaughter. Earlier that evening Mrs. Ellis had complained of pressure in her chest, so her daughter had brought her in to the emergency room. Mrs. Ellis told me what she hadn't told her daughter (because she hadn't wanted to worry her during her pregnancy): that during the past nine months she had had two open-heart operations back in St. Louis. I'd gotten an EKG on her, started an IV, hooked her up to oxygen, and was waiting for the backup cardiologist to give me a call.

On another bed I had a little old lady who, if they ever put out a casting call for someone to play Grandma Moses in the movies, would have walked away with the part hands down. She was seventy-seven years old, probably weighed about ninety pounds, and stood maybe half an inch over five feet tall. When she breathed, her lungs sounded like two strands of hair being rubbed together. Her three sons, brawny guys over six feet tall who might have been wrestlers, pro football players, or truck drivers, told me when they brought her in, "Ma's been awful wheezy lately." "Lately" turned out to be the last couple of weeks. "Ma" herself gave me the reason as to why she was so wheezy. Seemed she started feeling so pert about a month ago that she decided to throw all her medicines away. She didn't believe in medicine anyway, leastwise not the kind these newfangled doctors gave out in plastic shotgun pellets. Roots and herbs was what she believed in, but nobody gave out roots and herbs anymore. She looked up at me hopefully as if she thought I might have some tucked away in my pocket, but when I didn't come up with any, she ceased being interested in anything I might have to say. Unfortunately, those plastic shotgun pellets she had thrown away were what had been keeping her going and helping her feel so pert. Now she was slipping into congestive heart failure. Her wheezing was due to fluid backing up in her lungs, a result of the weak pumping action of her heart.

So she was another candidate for the backup cardiologist, who was taking his own sweet time about arriving. Until he did come, these two borderline cases were, of course, my responsibility.

And I kept having the feeling that things were going to get worse. That the other shoe was going to drop.

Which it did.

First a dour old gentleman with several fishhooks dangling from his left palm came through the doors, followed closely by Alice, who mumbled hurriedly, "The police are bringing in some woman..."

Now Alice is not usually a mumbler; she usually tells me precisely why the police are bringing someone in. I was going to ask her why they were bringing in "some woman," but she went right on talking before I could get in a single word.

"... and this is Mr. Plantich. He has—"

I was a little miffed, so I interrupted her. "Don't tell me, Alice. Let me guess."

"What?"

"He has nine fishhooks dangling from his left palm, right?"

Mark, who was standing nearby, guffawed.

Alice glared at him and then me, turned on her heel, and left.

As the doors at one end of the corridor swung shut behind her, those at the opposite end of the corridor opened and two policemen entered, supporting a woman between them. Sometimes that corridor has a definite Dante's Inferno feeling to it.

I left Mark to get Mr. Plantich settled on bed 5 while I hurried to talk to the police.

"What's wrong?" I asked, though I had the sinking feeling I already knew.

"She says she's been raped," one of the officers replied curtly.

I pointed toward the private examining room, then flagged Shirley down. I asked her to get the rape tray out and have the victim sign the consent form.

As I stood in the corridor for several moments, a whole plethora of thoughts troubled my mind—the kind that always assail me when I have to examine a rape victim—because rape is the kind of crisis that, more than any other, calls the emotions into play: mine, those of my staff, the police, and the victim.

With victims of other types of crises—heart attacks, automobile accidents, drug overdoses—I am concerned with restoring the physical well-being of the patient. With rape victims, I believe it is their psychological well-being that is often in greatest jeopardy. And yet the nature of the examination I have to give them and the kinds of questions I have to ask compel me, it seems, to jeopardize their emotional health even further.

After entering the examination room, the first thing the rape victim has to do is sign the following consent statement:

> I understand that hospitals and physicians are required by penal code section 11160–11161.5 to report to law enforcement authorities the name and whereabouts of any persons who are victims of sexual assault or who have suffered injuries inflicted by a deadly weapon or in violation of a penal law and the type and extent of those injuries. Knowing this, I consent to indicated treatment.
>
> ————————————————
> Patient or Parent or Guardian

The rape victim's signing such a statement accomplishes two things: It authorizes the EM physician to examine her and treat her injuries (sometimes *his*, but I'm going to use "her" and "she" throughout this discussion. Assaults by males upon males do occur, but they are far less frequent); and it identifies the woman—on a black-and-white printed form which will subsequently be given to the police—as the victim of a sexual assault.

I know that having the rape victim sign this form is necessary. I also know that being identified in this way is often disturbing to an already distraught person.

After the rape victim signs the form, she is given the option of signing a second consent statement—one that authorizes the examining physician to collect and preserve evidence of the assault. This statement reads as follows:

> I further understand that a separate medical examination for evidence of sexual assault at public expense can, with my consent, be conducted by the treating physician to discover and preserve evidence of the assault. If so conducted, the report of the examination and any evidence obtained will be released to law enforcement. Knowing this, I consent to a medical examination for evidence of sexual assault.
>
> _____
> Patient or Parent or Guardian

The rape victim does not have to sign, but the woman who wants her attacker arrested and convicted will do so, because it is only on the basis of such evidence that a conviction can take place.

I suppose it all sounds fairly simple: Examine the victim, collect the evidence.

Collecting the evidence to substantiate a rape, however, isn't easy.

The process begins with my subjecting the rape victim to a veritable barrage of questions—ones I find it difficult to ask a distraught patient. Here are some of the questions I am required to ask:

> Where did the rape take place? Were you in a bed, in a car, on the street?

If you were physically restrained, how were you physically restrained?

Describe the assault.

Do you know the name . . . or names . . . of your assailants? How many were there?

Was a weapon such as a gun or a knife used?

Was a foreign object used? If so, what was it, and where and how was it used?

What acts were committed? Coitus? Fellatio? Cunnilingus? Sodomy?

During the assault, was your vagina . . . or anus . . . penetrated? If so, how?

Did the assailant experience ejaculation? Vaginal? Oral? Anal? Other?

Did the assailant use a condom?

During the assault, did you vomit? Lose consciousness?

After the assault, what did you do? Wipe or wash yourself? Bathe? Douche? Vomit? Change your clothes? Brush your teeth? Urinate? Defecate?

It doesn't take a superactive imagination to envision the effect these kinds of questions may have upon a rape victim. Such questions essentially require the rape victim to relive her experience.

Prior to (or interspersed with) these questions I will also have to tell a rape victim that she may have contracted venereal disease as a result of the rape.

During the physical examination that follows the verbal interrogation, I will tell the rape victim exactly what I'm looking for and why. It seems to me that listening to me explain what I'm doing has to be easier for a woman than simply lying there in silence while I probe her already violated body.

I tell her I'm looking for lacerations, scratches, bruises, friction burns; in other words, signs of a physical attack. Often rape victims are in such a state of shock that they're unaware of physical wounds—even severe ones—they may have suffered. And evidence of a physical attack is important in a courtroom. It's one of the few things that lend a rape victim's accusations credibility. The typical attitude prevalent in the courtroom is reflected in a statement made not too long ago by a New York State assemblyman:

> When the defiled female says "That is the gentleman who raped me," we need corroboration. If her jaw is broken, for example, that is proof of force. Otherwise how do we know she was raped?

I tell the woman I have to comb through her pubic hair to see whether there are any "strange" hairs present. If there are, an attempt can be made to match such hairs with those of the suspected rapist.

When I examine the external pelvic and internal genital area, I explain that I'm looking for tears, cuts, bruises . . . again, signs of physical force. I'll ask the woman when her last menstrual period was, in an attempt to determine whether she is likely to be fertile. I'll ask her whether she uses an IUD or birth control pills. I'll ask her whether she is, or whether she thinks the possibility exists that she might be, pregnant.

And I have to tell rape victims that they might become pregnant as a result of the rape. (One out of a hundred rape victims does.)

I'll show the rape victim the speculum, the duck-billed instrument I will insert into the vagina in order to see the cervix and vaginal tract, where I will look for signs of recent intercourse. Most women have been examined with a speculum as part of routine gynecological examinations—most, but not all. So I never assume a woman has seen or even knows what a speculum is. I explain that live sperm can be found in the cervix for up to five days after intercourse. However, in the vagina, live sperm are usually found only up to six hours after intercourse. I will ask the woman when she last had "normal" intercourse. After taking a vaginal smear, I will remove the speculum. The physical examination is essentially finished. I then have a nurse administer a shot of penicillin to protect the victim from gonorrhea or syphilis. And finally, I discuss the options open to rape victims in case they become pregnant as a result of the rape.

If I feel the probability is high that the victim was fertile at the time of the rape, I will offer diethylstilbestrol (DES), a synthetic estrogenic substance, popularly known as the morning-after pill. Taking DES will disrupt a woman's hormonal balance, thereby probably—though not with 100 percent certainty—terminating pregnancy. There are possible side effects: Nausea and vomiting are the most common, but DES can also cause abdominal pain and distress, swelling and tenderness of the breasts, loss of appetite, diarrhea, weariness, tingling sensations, dizziness, headaches, depression, the appearance of purple blotches on the skin, and various allergic reactions. The drug may also aggravate conditions of epilepsy, migraine, asthma, and cardiac or renal dysfunction. DES is effective only if first administered within twenty-four hours of intercourse, and it must be taken for five consecutive days. Because of the nausea and vomiting, many women do not complete the five-day course. If DES doesn't work, the woman should have a D. and C. (dilation and curettage, dilating the cervix and scraping the uterus), since there is an increased chance of cancer to the unborn fetus. A woman's hormonal balance will correct itself fairly soon after she stops taking DES, though she may not have her menstrual period at its expected time.

Another option the rape victim has, if she does not want to take DES, is to wait and see if her menstrual period occurs within five to ten days of its expected time. If it does not, either a D. and C. or menstrual extraction may be done. Menstrual extraction is the removal of the uterine lining by suction through a very narrow tube inserted through the cervix. In many cases, the tube, or cannula, can be inserted without anesthetizing the patient or dilating the cervix. This procedure is faster than a D. and C., it is less complicated, and there is less risk of uterine perforation. Its only drawback is that it must be performed within five to ten days after menstruation is due.

As I have said, experiencing all of the above—the verbal interrogation, the physical examination, receiving the shot to prevent venereal disease, exploring the options in the event of pregnancy—is highly distressing to the rape victim. But having to be the instigator of such things is also unpleasant for the examining physician.

The emotional trauma a person has suffered as a result of a rape leaves that person in need of comfort and care. Yet that person's body, both externally and internally, immediately after the rape may well supply the most important legal evidence against the rapist if he comes to trial. And so the physician, in order to corroborate that a sexual assault has taken place, must become, in a sense, an adjunct of the law. (Rape, by the way, is a legal term, not a medical one.)

There's so damned much misunderstanding attached to rape, stuff that doesn't make sense, that shouldn't be part of our twentieth-century consciousness. I've discussed this with other doctors. It seems to be generally true that all the old Victorian beliefs—such as that rape only happens to women who provoke it; or that if a woman resists it's impossible to rape her—persist on some subliminal, emotional level. They manifest themselves in our initial reluctance to treat a rape victim, our sense of "dis-ease" when we do treat one; our relief when the episode is over. A lot of doctors say they don't want to treat rape victims because they don't want to become involved in lengthy court cases, but I doubt that that's the real reason. More often than not, attending physicians aren't even summoned into court, because the medical-record form filled out immediately after the rape occurred provides adequate evidence. I think the real reason lies in the mixed emotions with which doctors confront rape victims.

However, it isn't just the male doctors who experience such ambivalent feelings toward rape victims. Women do, too—women doctors and women nurses. And prosecutors have been known to say that women make terrible jurors during rape trials because it's often impossible to convince them that rape is not the victim's fault.*

And for men confronted by a rape victim: If a rape can be attributed to something the victim did, the male observer can

---

* June Bundy Csida and Joseph Csida, *Rape—How to Avoid It and What to Do About It If You Can't* (Chatsworth, Calif.: Books for Better Living, 1974), p. 43.

point the accusing finger at the female victim and relieve his own sex of responsibility.

Even rape victims themselves often view what has happened to them with a "victim" mentality. Many women have been culturally conditioned to be passive. The threat of violence can paralyze such a woman so that she can't even scream, let alone hit out at her attacker. But if a woman doesn't resist a rapist—and many women do not because they are in a state of frozen shock at the time and cannot; or because the rapist is holding a knife to their throat or a gun to their head and is threatening to use it— she feels guilty. A psychiatrist I once talked to described it as "the castle myth." The man is seen as the aggressor, the soldier laying siege to the castle. The woman is seen as the defender of the sacred treasure within the castle. If the man succeeds in forcing his way in and capturing the treasure, he has succeeded in his purpose. Far from feeling guilt or remorse, he simply feels that he did what he set out to do. The woman, however, experiences a sense of failure, because she has somehow allowed the treasure to be taken. She was not vigilant enough, brave enough, resourceful enough. She is the one who will be accused; she is the one who will be put on trial: Why was she hitchhiking? Why was she alone in a deserted place? Why was she out so late at night? Why did she open the door without knowing who it was?

I feel certain that's why so many women don't report rape (it's widely accepted that only one-fourth of the rapes that occur are ever reported); why women are unwilling to face the ordeal of the traditional rape trial.

If a "blame the victim" mentality underlies the stigma attached to rape, I hope I can do something in these pages to dispel it, simply by describing some of the rape victims I have treated in the emergency room.

Martha, for example, was a polio victim with matchstick-thin, lifeless legs who had been confined to a wheelchair for thirty-seven of her forty-three years. She was sitting in her wheelchair on her front porch one sunny Sunday afternoon. Her mother, who lived with her, had gone to visit a friend. A tall, muscular young man walking past her house saw her; turned abruptly into her yard; bounded up the steps to the porch, saying, "I'm gonna fuck you, I'm gonna fuck you"; whisked her out of her wheelchair, knocking it over in the process; carried her into the house, into a bedroom, threatening as he did so to "cut her tits off and stick them in her mouth" if she screamed; then raped her. A passerby who knew Martha noticed the overturned wheelchair and called the police.

Just last week I treated a young woman in her eighth month of pregnancy who had been assaulted by three men. One of the men became impotent when he saw her swollen abdomen, but the other two were neither disturbed nor deterred by her condition.

Six months ago I treated a seventy-four-year-old woman who had been raped.

Two months ago, a five-year-old child.

And a little over a month ago, I treated a woman who so stubbornly resisted her rapist that he banged her head up and down on the floor, causing her to lose consciousness and end up with a fractured skull.

Were these women, in any sense of the word, guilty of provoking the sexual assaults? Of course not.

I cite these cases simply to make the point that there are rapists out there who will rape a paralyzed woman in a wheelchair just as easily as they will a woman hitchhiking on a lonely road at night, that the motivating need, force, whatever you want to call it, lies within the rapist, not the victim.

In *Patterns in Forcible Rape*, Menachem Amir cites two categories of rapists: the "psychiatric" rapist and the "criminal" rapist. Amir states that the "psychiatric" rapist is sick, and knows it. He often has a higher than average IQ, may come from a wealthy background, and may have a high level of education. The "psychiatric" rapist will sometimes feel guilt and remorse after committing rape, but that won't stop him from committing rape again. On the other hand, the profile of the "criminal" rapist isn't significantly different from that of other felons convicted of robbery, burglary, and other types of assault. The "criminal" rapist is usually in his twenties, probably belongs to an ethnic minority, has a history of previous criminal activity, and is likely to have used alcohol or drugs prior to his crime. Either type will rape without provocation from the victim.

I think this is what has got to be understood once and for all. It is especially important today, when women in both their private and professional lives must take more risks than they ever have before—living alone, working alone, traveling alone. And the incidence of rape is escalating. In Los Angeles, for example, the number of reported rapes rose from 1,988 in 1970 to 2,062 in 1971 to 2,205 in 1972. In 1978 in Los Angeles County, there were 5,000 cases of rape referred to local law enforcement authorities. From these, 1,800 rapists were arrested. Complaints were filed against 400 of them by the district attorney's office, and 185 were convicted. That's a meager 3.5 percent of the 1,800 arrested. And Los Angeles boasts one of the highest conviction rates in the country.

Once when Israeli Prime Minister Golda Meir's all-male cabinet proposed a curfew on Israeli women to curb an outbreak of rapes, she answered, "But it's the men attacking the women. If there is to be a curfew, let the men stay home."

Think about that.

Currently, some things are being done to help rape victims. Not enough, but it's a start.

Rape crisis centers have been established in most metropolitan cities, staffed by paraprofessionals who have been trained to help rape victims cope with the scarring emotional trauma. And some hospitals have set up "chaplaincy" programs, wherein a number of clergy (male and female) have agreed to be on call to minister to rape victims in emergency rooms. Interestingly enough, participants in these programs have reported that the majority of rape victims are helped more by talking to male chaplains than to women. I suspect this is because the rape victim is extremely reluctant to discuss her ordeal with the significant males in her life—her husband or boyfriend, her father—and if she receives comfort, counsel, and understanding from male clergy, it helps her believe she may receive similar understanding from the significant males in her life.

Certainly doctors and policemen should be made aware of how important their attitude is when treating rape victims. When you realize that a woman who has been raped by a man usually has no recourse except to turn to other males (policemen and doctors) for help, and that her experience with that doctor or policeman has the potential of damaging or having a healing effect on her, wouldn't it make sense to have workshops for medical and law-enforcement personnel in which they would be taught how to minister to rape victims?

These were the kinds of thoughts that passed through my mind as I stood outside the examining room where a rape victim was waiting for me.

I wondered what her experience had been thus far with the police. The policeman I had spoken to had said, curtly, "She says she's been raped"; not simply, "She's been raped."

As I entered the examining room, Shirley handed me the signed consent form. I read it slowly. The victim's name was Sally Farran, and she was twenty-seven years old. She had signed both consent statements.

I looked up at her. Sally Farran had dark auburn hair pulled back into a bun; hazel eyes that wouldn't meet mine. Pale and nervous, she looked frightened as hell.

I told her I had to ask her some questions about what had happened, questions I knew would be distressing, but which I hoped she would do her best to answer. She did.

Sally was a schoolteacher. She lived alone in one of the numerous condominiums in the foothills. She had been getting ready for bed when she thought she heard a noise in her living room. She was positive she had locked her door, but she left her bedroom to investigate. As she entered the shadowy living room, a man—tall, husky, over six feet tall—grabbed her from behind, and with one hand squeezing her throat, told her she was dead if she screamed. Then he half pushed, half carried her into her bedroom, threw her down on the bed, and raped her. She was extremely frightened and did not resist.

She called the police after he left, though her assailant had told her he would come back and kill her if she did. The police had searched her neighborhood but had found no one answering the description she gave them of her attacker.

She wasn't certain she would press charges even if they did.

Sally was planning to be married next summer; her fiancé was an engineer working in another state. She definitely did not want him to know what had happened to her.

It was clear to me that she needed counseling. Most rape victims do. At the very least, they usually experience a crisis in their sex lives after being raped. For women who have had no previous sexual experience, the aftereffects are acute and long-lasting. For women who are sexually experienced, fear occurs when they attempt to resume normal sexual relationships. Some rape victims are able to return to normal sexual activity after about six weeks; others continue long after that to have grave difficulty in responding sexually to a man. Consequently, whether they initially intended to or not, rape victims usually end up telling their husbands or boyfriends what happened.

The husbands and boyfriends of rape victims I have talked to seem to be divided into two groups: one sympathetic and understanding; the other hostile and rejecting. The latter includes husbands who view their wives as pieces of property, as "chattel." When such a man's wife is raped, he feels his "possession" has been damaged and is therefore no longer of any value. He may even feel his wife is so tainted that he doesn't want to have anything further to do with her.

The rape victims themselves go through several phases of a reaction pattern called the "rape-trauma syndrome." During the first, most acute phase, while the victim's body heals itself, the woman is almost constantly afraid of being alone. This phase usually diminishes in intensity after two to three weeks. The second phase begins when the woman starts to reorganize her life. Nightmares and phobias are common at this time. In addition, the woman may have headaches, stomachaches, backaches, and urinary-tract reactions. However, the longest-lasting problems arise with the emotional aftereffects that manifest themselves throughout the third phase. These range from fear, humiliation, and embarrassment to rage, anger, and a wish for revenge, but the most destructive are self-blame and guilt.

I try to persuade all the rape victims I treat to seek help from a rape crisis center. Staff members at the center are skilled in helping rape victims overcome their trauma. They provide counseling, arrange contact with other women who have been raped and are willing to talk about it, make referrals to professionals for psychotherapy should it become necessary, and inform the rape victim about court procedures and tactics used by defense lawyers should the rapist be brought to trial.

At the end of my examination, Sally Farran agreed to let Shirley call the rape crisis center on her behalf.

As I left Sally and walked out into the corridor, Gloria informed me that the backup cardiologist had arrived to treat my two heart patients. That meant that the only patient left for me to worry about was the man on bed 5 with the fish hooks dangling from his palm.

The sour expression on his face as I rounded the curtain let me know he felt he'd been kept waiting much too long.

"Sorry to be so long," I said brusquely. "Let me see that hand."

Wordlessly he extended his hand, palm upward.

I gave him a shot of Novocain to numb his palm, then set about disengaging the eight fish hooks from the ninth one, imbedded in his palm. "How are you set for tetanus?"

"Had booster shots in the army fifteen years ago," he replied. "Nothing since then."

"Well, a booster shot is good for at least five years and probably more, but I wouldn't push it to fifteen," I said. "Only a hundred Americans got tetanus last year, but half of those who got it died. So I'm going to order a half cc of tetanus toxoid for you."

He nodded. "Okay. Say, Doc . . ."

"Hm?"

"What'd she do?"

I frowned. "Who?"

"The woman who was raped. I heard the police talking about her out in the corridor while I was waiting. Was she hitchhiking, or drunk, or what?"

I know I shouldn't have answered him. Questions like that don't deserve answers. But as I pushed the fish-hook barb through his skin, cut it off, then pulled the hook back through the other way, minus the barb, I thought about what he had asked, and it got under *my* skin.

"Well, I'll tell you what she did," I said. "She drove home from the school where she teaches, went into her apartment, cooked her dinner, then got ready for bed."

"Yeah, yeah," he said. "Go on."

"That's it," I said.

He stared at me, then shook his head. "She didn't tell you the whole story," he said finally. "The guy must've had some reason. She just didn't tell you everything."

"You're probably right," I said. "She probably didn't tell me everything. She couldn't. Only the rapist could do that."

12

Diatribes and Digressions

THE EMERGENCY ROOM is the only open door for large numbers of people who perceive themselves to be in a state of medical crisis.

Once upon a time, general practitioners treated many of the patients now seen by EM physicians. But general practitioners are dwindling in number, and those who remain tend to practice medicine within the same nine-to-five framework as the rest of America's doctors. The things that GPs did in their midnight visits to patients' homes in the first half of this century are now either done by the EM physician or they're not done at all.

Perhaps it is our accessibility to all patients who come to the doors of the emergency room that differentiates EM physicians from the rest of the nation's doctors. We are a breed apart, because it is an inherent aspect of our profession that we will see anyone at any time. And most Americans know this—know that should they need to see a doctor, one is available to them in the local emergency room.

Inevitably I think it is this accessibility to the general population that shapes the way EM physicians view the world. We see all kinds of people—rich and poor, old and young, infirm and healthy, the oppressed and the oppressors—at their worst and at their best. We also see other doctors at their worst and at their best and see ourselves at our worst and our best. Because another thing that distinguishes us from other doctors is that we must be ready, at any time while we are on duty, to treat a patient on the verge of death. And sometimes they come in twos, threes, fours—from highway accidents, from urban disasters. Once you've been through that—having to leave the side of someone who is probably dying to tend to someone who will certainly die if you don't do something—you don't forget it. Somewhere inside, in some hidden place, you learn to maintain a constant readiness to confront disaster.

Being forced to deal constantly with crises breeds, I think, a certain intolerance for things that negate the quality of life: waste; indifference; apathy. It certainly breeds intolerance for abuses of the medical profession.

I have already vented my feelings about on-call doctors who manage not to be available—or, if they are available, respond in a reluctant, sludgelike fashion that can and sometimes does imperil the lives of patients. Another subject I feel I cannot close this book without commenting on is how the welfare system in this country both abuses and is abused by the medical profession.

The welfare system itself is, of course, founded upon negative factors: social inequality, lack of educational opportunity, unemployment, poor housing, abject poverty. And it is a fact of life that poverty contributes to and often culminates in sickness: alcoholism, mental instability, dependence on drugs. So many of the patients we see in the emergency room are people on welfare that we inevitably begin to have some very strong feelings about the welfare system itself.

I wish I could say I have never had a hostile thought toward anyone on welfare, anyone less fortunate than I, but I can't. Too often I get the feeling that welfare patients I treat believe that because I'm a doctor I'm guilty of economic oppression. And it's hard not to respond in kind to patients who are hostile and resentful. But I had to struggle like hell to become a doctor, and I don't think I should be blamed for it.

Perhaps the most frustrating attitude I encounter is indifference. So many people seem to care less about themselves than I care about them. They don't keep appointments for follow-up visits, they don't follow instructions, if they run out of medicine they don't come back to get more. When I try to put myself into their shoes I realize that retreat into apathy must at times seem to be the only viable solution to their problems. But all of my training and all of my instincts cause me to reject this solution. I don't want them to be apathetic; I want them to *want* to get well.

And then there are the doctors who feed off the medical-care system engendered by apathy: Medicaid. Most competent doctors abhor Medicaid, for several reasons. Primary among these are (1) the government decides how much it will pay for given medical procedures—and the amounts it pays are not equitable; they are substantially lower than what private insurance carriers pay; (2) payments take anywhere from six to eighteen months to reach the doctors who provide the medical services for Medicaid patients; and (3) the government requires three times as much paperwork for Medicaid patients as private insurance carriers require for their patients.

When there are factors inherent in a governmental medical-care system that alienate the doctors who are the providers of medical care, that system becomes vulnerable to incompetence and abuse.

There is a pecking order in medicine just as in every other profession. Once upon a time, prior to the 1960s, emergency room physicians were at the bottom of the pecking order. They were the moonlighters of the profession—the too old or too young, the alcoholic or the infirm—doctors who didn't have anywhere else to practice.

No more. Now doctors who specialize in Medicaid patients are at the bottom of the pecking order.

Who are the Medicaid doctors? Some of them are young doctors just out of medical school, just getting started in practice, who may have put themselves in debt to finance their studies and can therefore barely afford to open an office. For these doctors, treating patients whose bills are paid eighteen months late is preferable to treating no patients at all. However, as these young doctors gradually become established in their communities, they begin to weed out their Medicaid patients.

Other Medicaid doctors are foreign medical graduates, FMGs, many of whom haven't mastered the English language. In some cases their training may not be as good as that of American doctors. While initially their financial expectations may not be as high as those of American doctors, once they begin to get established and learn "the American way," they too become increasingly reluctant to see welfare patients.

So, after the newly graduated, impoverished doctors, and after the FMGs, what's left? Institutions called health maintenance organizations (HMOs) often referred to by other doctors, including me, as welfare mills.

Envision, if you will, Medicaid as a giant bureaucratic shark, and doctors operating HMOs as the remora fish who suck on it.

The original theory behind Health Maintenance Organizations was that by having a certain number of subscribers prepay a medical-care fee to a physician group, the cost of medical care to the individual could be kept down. This theory did not take into account the profit motive of the individuals who own and operate many Health Maintenance Organizations. These individuals know that one way they can increase their profits is by increasing the number of people who subscribe to their HMO. And one way to increase the number of subscribers is to hire "hawkers" to go from door to door to sign people up, paying these hawkers a finder's fee for every person they enroll. Hawkers—with finders' fees dangling in front of their noses—have been known to mislead people about what services HMOs actually provide.

The individuals who own and operate Health Maintenance Organizations know that another way they can increase their profits is by getting themselves the equivalent of a government subsidy. For an HMO, the equivalent of a government subsidy is patients on welfare. HMO operators reason that they can make money on welfare patients by seeing more patients faster. The criterion by which the government measures the efficacy of HMOs is quantity, not quality. The government pays for the number of tonsils removed, not for how well they are removed; nor is any attempt made to determine whether or not they should have been removed in the first place.

HMOs further increase their profits by staffing their organizations with new medical graduates who can't yet afford to open their own offices, or with FMGs anxious to get a foothold in the United States. They pay them twenty to thirty dollars an hour, and see that they generate forty to sixty dollars an hour in business.

Still another way HMOs increase profits is to have their doctors work a rigid eight-hour day with a minimal amount of equipment. Any patient who needs to be seen outside that eight hours, or who needs a special test, can be sent to—you guessed it—the emergency room. And if an HMO patient gets in trouble, takes too many sleeping pills—for example, pills that never should have been prescribed in the first place—you know where that patient ends up: the emergency room.

HMO doctors aren't the only abusers of the welfare system. There is a certain breed of lawyer who preys on it as well, a type I call "malpractice artists." In California, 10 percent of the population is on welfare. Fifty percent of the state's malpractice cases come from this 10 percent of the population, thanks to the malpractice artists.

Here's how it works. Malpractice artists seek out welfare patients who are receiving medical care and, when the circumstances seem right, convince them to sue their doctors. These malpractice artists know that the insurance companies that provide malpractice insurance want to avoid litigation of comparatively small claims because (1) their own legal staff is limited; and (2) since verdicts are sometimes rendered on emotional rather than judicial grounds, the possibility of losing a case always exists, no matter what the circumstances. The malpractice artist defends the welfare patient on a contingency basis, charging nothing if the patient loses, but keeping half of the award if he wins. And chances are, the insurance company will elect to make an out-of-court settlement for five to ten thousand dollars regardless of whether the doctor involved is innocent or guilty. The lawyer keeps half the money, the patient gets the other half. Who loses? Ultimately, the public, which pays the cost whenever malpractice insurance goes up.

You know what it would take to abolish over half the malpractice suits in America today? The abolition of the contingency system. America is the only country in the world that permits a contingency system. Why we tolerate its existence, I cannot fathom. It's a system that literally spawns leeches.

The malpractice artists aren't the only ones who leech off it. There's another group it galls me even to write about—Personal Injury System operators: P.I.S. men. These are doctors and lawyers who work together. They have tow truck operators, ambulance drivers, nurses, and orderlies working for them as "finders." When an accident occurs, say, in a shopping center, the tow truck driver or ambulance attendant who is called to the scene refers the injured person to a P.I.S. lawyer or doctor (and later collects a finder's fee of one or two hundred dollars cash for doing so). The P.I.S. doctor treats the patient over a period of several months. Often, this doctor will send the patient to an orthopedist or neurologist for special examinations and tests, making certain the patient runs up a bill of several thousand dollars. The P.I.S. lawyer then files a claim with the insurance company, together with lengthy medical reports corroborating an injury that may be minor in severity but is exceedingly complex in presentation. The insurance company, faced with hundreds of claims like this and a limited number of lawyers of its own, would rather pay the claim than risk a long and possibly costly court battle. The doctor's bill is paid. The lawyer gets his contingency fee, usually 50 percent of the settlement. The patient receives three to six thousand dollars. So, who loses? Again, the public. Think about it the next time you pay your insurance premium.

I deeply resent a system that nurtures malpractice artists, that nurtures a Personal Injury System. Inevitably it affects the way I practice my profession. If I get hauled into court by some shyster lawyer trying to leech off a welfare patient's misery, it affects my attitude toward all the welfare patients I see. It increases the time and effort I expend trying to "cover my ass" when I could be doing other, better things with my time—like researching new techniques that I could use to better care for my patients.

Anyone thinking about entering any of the medical specialties—be it emergency medicine or any other—should know that the divorce rate is high. Being a doctor is a physically demanding and emotionally taxing profession. The spiritual rewards medicine offers are proportionate to however much of the self a person is willing to expend.

Emergency medicine, like any other medical specialty, isn't

as accessible to the physician just out of medical school as it once was. At one time, if a physician wanted to be a specialist in, say, pediatrics, all he had to do was voluntarily limit his practice to children, and spend five dollars for a plaque proclaiming that he was a pediatrician. Now, of course, he must go through a period of residency and a whole examination/certification process.

A similar change has taken place in emergency medicine during the last few years. Once, almost any doctor could work in an emergency room. Now a residency, or a certified period of practical experience, and an examination/certification process are required.

The more specialized the medical profession becomes, the more one specialty is insulated from another. This has its drawbacks, because a given specialist tends to look at one particular kind of tree and lose track of the existence of any other kind, let alone ever cast an eye at the entire forest. But it also has its advantages: A specialist tends to master all the fine points of his or her specialty and can keep abreast of all the latest developments in it.

The specialties of emergency medicine and family practice mandate that doctors keep their eyes on the forest. I like looking at that forest. And, as I stated before, I like the fact that an emergency medicine physician doesn't have to maintain an office or cope with personnel, billing, or governmental rules and regulations.

The hospital I work in takes 25 percent of the gross billing generated by the emergency room in return for providing space and equipment, doing the accounts, and so on. It also pays the cost of my malpractice insurance. The policy covering the physician group of which I am a member costs the hospital $3,500 per month. This amount is deducted from the gross billing generated by the emergency room, so it ultimately comes out of each patient's pocket. Figuring 23,000 patients per year, that works out to roughly $1.85 per patient.

Which brings us to the question: How much can you earn if you decide to become an EM physician?

Well, a few hospitals hire their own emergency medicine

physicians and pay them a flat salary that can range anywhere from forty thousand dollars to seventy thousand dollars.

Some emergency medicine physicians belong to small physician groups that have been contracted to staff the emergency room of a given hospital.

Most EM physicians work for large physician groups that staff the emergency rooms of several hospitals. The EM physicians who work for physician groups work as independent contractors paid on an hourly basis, anywhere from twenty to sixty dollars an hour.

The whole subject of physician groups is certainly something the young would-be EM physician must be aware of because chances are, unless the physician contracts to work with a physician group, he or she won't be able to work in an emergency room.

Physician groups exist in almost all the specialties. Outside the hospital, cardiologists, gastroenterologists, oncologists, and obstetrician-gynecologists practice together in private office settings.

Inside the hospital, pathologists, radiologists, and anesthesiologists practice in groups within the hospital setting. In fact, physician groups in these essential in-hospital specialties may contract to provide services for more than one hospital.

The same thing is now true of emergency medicine physicians. With one difference. The above-mentioned specialists operate their own groups and share equally in the profits. Groups of EM physicians tend to be run by owner/operators who "skim" a percentage off the top. "Skimmers" usually staff the emergency rooms of several hospitals. Some "skimmers" staff the emergency rooms of hospitals in several states. The contracts negotiated with hospitals by these "skimmers" can take many forms. Hospitals may pay a set fee to have their emergency room staffed, or the "skimmers" may take a percentage of the gross billings generated by the emergency room.

The primary factor the fledgling EM physician must be aware of is that there is a large profit motive operating among these "skimmers," just as there is among the HMOs. "Skimmers" invariably end up living in "fat city."

For example: Say an average, run-of-the-mill hospital is willing to pay $10,000 a month—or $120,000 a year—to have its emergency room staffed 24 hours per day, 365 days a year.

One doctor couldn't staff that emergency room alone—not even for $120,000 a year.

So the hospital administrator is likely to go to the operator of a physician group.

The operator of the group, himself an M.D., has emergency medicine physicians working for him as "independent contractors," which means they pay their own Social Security tax, unemployment tax, health insurance, pension funds, and so on. All the operator of the physician group has to pay is an hourly fee for their services. But before he pays his doctors anything, the operator of a physician group takes a percentage off the top for what he calls "administrative costs." "Administrative costs" might include putting on educational programs for doctors; running CPR courses for nurses and paramedics; wining and dining the administrative staff of a hospital; or, it might not include much of anything. The percentage skimmed off the top for "administrative costs" usually runs between 10 and 20 percent.

So, let's take the hospital that was willing to pay $10,000 per month to have its emergency room staffed. The "administrative cost" skimmed off the top of that would be $1000–$2000 per month.

An enterprising physician group operator, or skimmer, will have a number of physicians working for him as independent contractors to staff the emergency rooms of several hospitals. Predicate ten hospitals. That would give a physician group operator $10,000–$20,000 per month possibly for not doing one hell of a lot.

Physician-group operators should not be allowed to do this. I think it amounts to fee splitting, which is illegal. A similar situation plagued radiology-physician groups until the American Board of Radiologists put a stop to it.

The American College of Emergency Physicians was only formally recognized by the AMA in 1979. And a lot of its officers happen to be operators of physician groups. As yet the ACEP hasn't taken any moral or ethical stand on the issue. But someday I think it will, and when it does, "skimming" will cease.

You may be wondering where the operators of physician groups find doctors who are willing to work for them. The same place the welfare mills find their doctors.

Take your average medical school graduate. After eight years of college, he or she received $6000 to $12,000 per year during internship, and $10,000 to $20,000 per year during residency. Then the operator of a physician group comes along and offers $40,000 to $60,000 a year to start, and it sounds too good to be true. Young doctors just out of school are willing to work hard, including holiday shifts, and to pay the group operator a percentage of their earnings. But after one or two years all doctors should receive a fair share of what the group operator actually earns.

Granted, even if a doctor works only a day or two a week for a group, he or she can earn a tidy sum.

Some hospitals with "slow" emergency rooms ("slow" meaning you will probably only see twenty-five to thirty patients, and most of these will be easy: flu, sprained ankles, and so on) are staffed by doctors working twenty-four-hour shifts. Probably your immediate reaction is that no doctor can work a twenty-four-hour shift and continue to be effective. But if a doctor is taking naps between patients, he or she can. Now. Say you're trying to open your own office. You decide to work one twenty-four-hour shift per week, and the operator of the physician group pays you twenty to twenty-five dollars per hour. For that one twenty-four-hour shift per week, you'll end up with $24,960 to $31,200 a year.

When I was starting out, I used to fly to Las Vegas from Los Angeles, which took two hours, work in a hospital there for from 48 to 72 hours at $22 per hour three or four times per month, and earn myself $1056–$1584 each time I did it. Not bad. But I worked for my money. The operators of physician groups don't do what I call work for their money. That's what rankles.

Maybe if enough new doctors coming into the profession are made aware of the situation, pressure can be brought to bear on the American College of Emergency Physicians to put a stop to this kind of thing. Many emergency medical corporations now service 100 or more hospital contracts over several states. Big money and big profits are involved, and the temptation to make emergency medicine into simply a business—with no professional identity—is great.

Another aspect of being an EM physician that newcomers to the profession need to know about is the difference between what hospital administrators say emergency rooms do and what they actually do.

Until very recently, hospital administrators seemed convinced that emergency rooms were nothing but trouble for a hospital; that they brought into the hospital undesirable people who never paid their bills; that the emergency room was an economic drain upon a hospital, a loser.

Let's take a closer look at what really goes on.

There is no question but that emergency care is expensive. Making highly skilled personnel available around the clock to see patients on an unscheduled, nonselective basis costs a fair amount of money.

But let's look at what the emergency medicine physician accomplishes, both on behalf of the patient and on behalf of the hospital.

On behalf of the patient: Insurance companies have been quick to realize that the twenty-four-hour availability of emergency medicine physicians can and does decrease the cost of medical care to the patient. Take the man who wakes up at 3 A.M. with chest pain, for example. He doesn't know whether or not he's having a heart attack. He goes to the emergency room. The emergency medicine physician administers one hundred dollars' worth of tests to determine whether or not the pain is indeed cardiac in nature. If it is, the man is admitted into the cardiac care unit of the hospital; if it isn't, he is sent home. If there was no emergency medicine physician on duty, patients with obscure chest pain in the middle of the night would be routinely admitted to the cardiac care unit and be charged ten times as much for a three-day stay there as they would for diagnostic procedures performed by the emergency medicine physician.

On behalf of the hospital: Hospitals use traditional cost-accounting methods to calculate how much it costs them to maintain an emergency room. They tally up the cost of the space, the equipment, and the high-salaried personnel, and balance it against the "emergency room fee" charged each patient who uses its services. What they don't take into account is the impact the existence of the emergency room has upon the hospital, both tangible and intangible.

Tangibly, the emergency room brings into greater usage the ancillary services of the hospital: respiratory therapy, the lab, EKG technicians, the pharmacy. These ancillary services are high-profit centers for a hospital. Typically, two-thirds of the bill the patient pays for a visit to the emergency room is for such services, yet the emergency room is never credited with generating the usage of these services. With their traditional accounting methods, hospitals credit the ancillary services themselves for generating this revenue.

Also tangibly, the emergency room acts as a point of entry for patients admitted into the hospital. Approximately 10 to 15 percent of the patients treated in emergency rooms are subsequently admitted to the hospital. An average patient admission will gross a hospital about two thousand dollars. However, since patients admitted via emergency rooms are usually more seriously ill than routine elective hospital admissions, these patients are therefore apt to utilize a greater number of diagnostic and therapeutic services. Consequently, their hospital stay will probably gross more than two thousand dollars for the hospital.

Intangibly, the emergency room is the window through which the majority of the public views its hospitals. The hospital where I work sees about 23,000 patients a year, and 2.6 persons accompanied these 23,000 patients to the hospital. Thus, over 80,000 persons gained an impression of the hospital from their visit to the emergency room.

So—far from being a drain on a hospital's resources—the emergency room is one of its lifelines.

The simplest, most objective way to analyze the impact the emergency room has on any given hospital would be to shut down the emergency room for a specified period of time, then calculate the resulting loss of revenue.

I suspect the results would be startling to even the most traditional hospital administrator.

I exhort you would-be EM physicians out there to remember these things. And if you do decide to join the ranks of those of us who staff hospital emergency rooms, and when budget time comes around and your hospital administrator denies you a new piece of equipment you sorely need, saying your department doesn't generate enough revenue, you'll know precisely what to say.

Epilogue

SOMETIMES IT'S HARD for me to remember how—once upon a time—I didn't know who I was, or even who I wanted to be. It was only a couple of decades ago, but it seems like light-years.

I was a lightweight then: no job I cared about; no commitment to meaningful personal relationships.

Now I have a profession that fulfills me, a wife I cherish, three kids I love, two Siamese cats, twenty-two goldfish, and a golden retriever named Sam.

I want to tell you about an incident involving Sam that happened a month or so ago. Sam got sick in the middle of the night. I called my vet's number and received a tape-recorded message telling me Dr. Bigelow would be in at 8 A.M., and that if my pet needed emergency care to call the emergency veterinarian service. And the number of the emergency service was given.

I called the number and was told to bring Sam right on down to the emergency room.

A pleasant admitting clerk took down all of Sam's vital statistics, then ushered us into a room where a veterinarian was waiting to see us. He examined Sam thoroughly, then told me Sam had contracted a fast-acting bacteria. He gave Sam a shot of penicillin and told me to take Sam in to see Dr. Bigelow the next morning.

I really liked the young doctor who treated Sam. He was efficient, intelligent, compassionate. Dr. Bigelow, I knew, was approaching retirement. So I asked the likable young doctor if he practiced as a veterinarian during the daytime in an office.

He said he didn't—that practicing as an emergency room veterinarian let him live the kind of life he wanted. He saw all kinds of cases during the twelve hours he was on duty, from 8 P.M. to 8 A.M. Some animals he brought back to life right from death's door. And when he went home in the morning, his time was his own.

I listened to what he had to say, and started to chuckle. I knew just what he meant.

Glossary

bag-breathing A temporary method of breathing for a patient who is having difficulty breathing or is not breathing at all. It is a soft rubber bag called an ambu bag that is hand-held and squeezed, thereby pushing out oxygen into the patient's lungs.

biocom A two-way radio used when communicating with paramedics in the field. It is hooked up to telemetry so that EKGs can be sent to the hospital to be read.

Bird machine A breathing device to which a patient is hooked up after an endotracheal tube is put down his throat or a nasotracheal tube into his lungs. The machine can alter the rate, depth, pressure, and percentage of oxygen the patient breathes. There are more sophisticated machines in use. Patients can remain on these machines for years. Karen Quinlan was on such a machine.

BUN Blood Urea Nitrogen. A lab measurement used by a physician as an indicator of how the kidneys are functioning.

CBC Complete Blood Count. For the lab, this means a hematocrit, a hemoglobin, and an actual count of 100 white cells from a peripheral smear of blood into the many different classes of white cells.

Code Blue A system used for brevity and secrecy in many hospitals to indicate to personnel that a patient's heart has stopped; i.e., cardiac arrest. The hospital intercom will announce, "Code Blue, room 318 . . . Code Blue, room 318" and certain predesignated personnel will respond.

Code 2, 3 A system used by police and ambulance to indicate how fast to respond to a call for assistance. Code 2 means as fast as possible; code 3 means to add lights and sirens.

CVP line Central Venous Pressure. An IV plastic flexible tube is threaded through a large needle in the neck directly into the right side of the patient's heart to enable the physician to measure the pressure in the right side of the heart. Various fluids and medications can be administered through the tubing and blood may also be drained from this same tube.

D5W Dextrose 5 percent in water or a 5 percent water solution of sugar.

flow sheet A sheet of paper on which various values such as temperature, blood pressure, heart rate, urinary output, and lab values are plotted against time. The patient's progress can be understood at a glance.

gurney A high bed with wheels, used to examine patients and push them from place to place in the hospital.

hemostat clamp A small surgical device used to grab and clamp blood vessels to control and stop bleeding.

IM Intramuscular, usually referring to how medication is given by needle.

IV Intravenous, giving a solution or medication directly into a vein.
otoscope An instrument for inspecting the ear. *Oto* means ear.
saline *Saline* means salt. A saline IV, or "normal saline," is a solution of salt and water that has the identical concentration of the salt in the blood. If a person is dehydrated, he is given just this, while if a person has lost blood, he receives normal saline to raise or maintain his blood pressure until he can be given blood. One can stick an IV in the patient within seconds and give him a saline solution, while to get the blood typed and crossmatched takes at least forty-five minutes, often longer. The saline solution comes in different concentrations and has different functions.

scoop and run A slang term used by ambulance and paramedics when they "scoop" the patient or victim up in a stretcher without any stabilization or treatment at the scene and "run" into the emergency room. This occurs mostly when the patient is severely injured and is near death.

stat Abbreviation for *immediately*, from the Latin word *statim*.

ten-four Part of a system used for brevity by the police and ambulance over the two-way radio; it means "message acknowledged."

Index

abdomen: nonpenetrating wounds to, 74; trauma to, 73–75. *See also* entries *under* "abdominal"
abdominal bleeding, diagnosis of, 77–78
abdominal distention, 84–85
abdominal muscles, rigidity of, 86, 91–93
abdominal pain, diagnosis of causes of, 80–97
abdominal X-rays, 88–89; swallowed objects and, 48
abortion, rape victims and, 193
accidents, 54–78; as cause of death, 5; diagnosis of injuries from, 69–71; with fish hooks, 188; and multiple injuries, 57–63; police and, 167; and pregnancy, 75–76; sexual, 99–100. *See also* head injuries
admitting clerk, role of, 14, 16–17, 57
adrenalin, 44, 108–9, 110
Against Medical Advice (AMA) form, 100, 166
age, diagnosis of abdominal pain and, 81, 88
airway obstructions, 35–36, 58–59, 106–7
alcoholics, 95–96, 167, 168–69, 173, 181–82
alligator forceps, 31, 49
ambu bag, 37

ambulance attendants, 2. *See also* paramedics
anaphylactic shock, 47
angel dust. *See* PCP
angina pain, 19–20
angiography, 27
animal bites, 63–65
ankle, broken or sprained, 72–73
answering services, physicians', 130–31
antibiotics, 111–12, 148
anticlotting drugs, 27
appendicitis, 81, 82, 83–84
aspirin, baby and adult, 111
asthma, 104–5, 108–10
athletic coaches, X-rays ordered by, 72–73
automatic breathing machines, 37–38. *See also* Bird machine

barbiturates, 154
barium enema, 94, 96–97
biocom calls, 7, 23–25, 32–34, 91, 120–22
Bird machine, 126, 152–53
bladder, burst, 75
bleeding: and hypovolemic shock, 46; and initial hematocrit, 69–70; internal, 77–78; intraabdominal, 69; and MAST suit, 62; undefined source of, 184–86. *See also* blood

blood: in stool or vomitus, 88, 93; typing and crossmatching, 60–61, 65, 124, 170
blood-alcohol tests, 56, 167
blood clots. *See* epidural hemorrhage; pulmonary embolism; subdural blood clot
blood-gas studies, 26–27, 45, 116, 126, 153
blood pressure, 58–59, 60, 66, 153, 171. *See also* vital signs
blood tests, 22, 113
bowel sounds, 75, 86–87
brain. *See* brain death; head injuries
brain death, diagnosis of, 45
breast implants, 180–81
breathing problems. *See* airway obstructions; asthma; hemothorax; upper-airway obstruction
broken neck, 125
broken ribs, 79–81, 83; and abdominal injuries, 75; cardiac compression and, 35; dangers of, 89–90, 94–95; hemothorax and, 59; kidney damage and, 70, 75; and maneuvers to open airway, 108
bullet wounds, 73, 146–48, 169–72
bystanders: and airway obstruction victims, 106; and seizure victims, 129–30

"cafe coronary," 107–8
call list of doctors, medical emergencies and, 8, 28–30, 48, 63, 65–66, 124, 126–27, 130–31, 188, 203
cancer, diagnosis of, 96–97, 176
cardiac arrest, 33–48, 109, 167–72
cardiac monitor, 15–16, 24, 33, 40, 41–42
cardiogenic shock, 46–47
cardiopulmonary resuscitation (CPR), 34–46, 51–52
C.A.T. scan, 143, 144
charcoal and magnesium slurry, 155, 158
chest pain: of angina, 19–20; diagnosis of causes, 12–13, 15–17, 24. *See also* cardiac arrest; heart attacks
chest-wall syndromes, 12

chest X-rays, 116, 153, 171
child abuse, 176–80
children: and accidents, 66; artificial ventilation of, 36; behavior in emergency room, 68; and cardiopulmonary resuscitation, 43; and external cardiac compression, 35; and facial lacerations, 140; genital injuries in, 22–23, 70–71; objects in ears of, 30–31; raped, 196; and skull fractures, 131; sore throats in, 110–12; subdural blood clots in, 141–44; and ticks, 136–38; urinary output measures in, 46. *See also* child abuse; infants; parents
Code Blue. *See* cardiac arrest
colon: cancer of, 94; penetrating wounds of, 73–74
colostomy, 74
congestive heart failure, 187–88
consciousness, level of, hypoxia and, 122–23
Consent to Treat forms, 16–17, 57, 181–82, 189–90
contingency system, 206–7
county hospitals, transfers to, 29, 47, 56, 65–66, 158–59, 166, 168–69
craniotomy, 140
cricothyrotomy, 108

death, causes of, 5, 13–14, 65, 114, 151–52
D. and C., rape victims and, 193
"decorticate positioning," 130
defibrillation paddles, 42–43, 183
deliveries in emergency room, 101–3
DES, rape victims and, 193
diagnosis: ambulance crew and, 24; incorrect, 6. *See also individual disorders*
dog bites, 63–65
Dopamine, 45, 46
drowning. *See* near-drownings
drug addicts, police attitude toward, 173
drug-overdose victims, *xi–xii*, 154; aggressive, 156–60; friends of, 166; induced vomiting in, 154–55; male-female differences in, 149–50; sui-

cide and, 149–52. *See also* hallucinogens
drug reactions, 18
drunken drivers, 56, 181–82. *See also* blood-alcohol tests

eardrum, perforation of, 134–36
ears: bleeding from, 134–36; fly in, 48–49; objects in, 30–31
earwax, purpose of, 30
Echoencephalograms, 143, 144
ectopic pregnancy, 81
elderly patients: and adrenalin, 108–9; cardiopulmonary resuscitation of, 44; external cardiac compression in, 35; intravenous insertion in, 39–40; police attitude toward, 174–75; poverty and, 93, 175–76
electric shock, cardiopulmonary resuscitation and, 42–43, 45
electrocardiogram (EKG), 17, 19, 21, 24, 70
electrocardiogram technicians, 17, 20
emergency medical technicians: role of, 2, 114, 133, 157–58, 162–66; salaries of, 14
emergency medicine: cost of, 212–13; growth as specialty, 1–14; specialization in, 207–11
emergency medicine physicians: earnings of, 208–11; emotional involvement with patients, 9–10, 52–53, 151; family life of, 10–11; relations with families of patients, 9, 21–22, 23, 51–53, 90–91, 111–12, 122; relations with police, 167–86; relations with private physicians, 22, 27–28, 94–95; relations with staff, 25, 41, 116–19, 124–25; and "skimmers," 209–11; typical shift of, 10, 14–22
emergency rooms: busy times, 6–7, 104; and cost of medical care, 212; description of, 7, 14; staff of, 7, 14, 132
endotracheal intubation, xi, xii, 37–39, 152–53, 170, 171
enemas, 113–14, 116–17
epidural blood clot, 141

epidural hemorrhage, 121–27, 128–29, 131–32
epilepsy, 129
erections, traumatic rupture of spinal cord and, 171. *See also* priapism
external cardiac compression, 34–35
eye injuries, from radiation or ultraviolet rays, 137

facial lacerations, plastic surgery for, 140
families of patients, 55–56, 127; behavior of, 15, 156–57; emotional involvement with, 52–53; and length of cardiopulmonary resuscitation efforts, 43–44; relations with emergency medicine physician, 9, 21–22, 30–31, 90–91, 131–32
fibrillation, 42–43
Foley catheter, 45–46, 124, 126, 170; plugged, 128
food, inhaled, 107–8
foreign medical graduates (FMGs), Medicaid patients and, 204–5
foreign objects: in ears, 48–49; in rectum, 97–99; swallowed, 48, 49–51. *See also* upper-airway obstruction
fractured skull, 131

gallbladder disease, 81, 82
gallstone, in small intestine, 91
gastric ulcer, perforated, 81, 82, 85, 92–93
gastrointestinal problems, 13, 48, 49–51, 96
general practitioners, decrease in number of, 5, 202

hallucinogens, 160, 161–66
head injuries, 132–34; craniotomy and, 140; and epidural hemorrhage, 121–27, 128–29, 131–32; gunshot wounds, 146–48; holes in skull, 132–34; scalp lacerations, 138–39; seizures from, 128–30; and skull X-rays, 143, 144–46; and spinal taps, 143–44; and subdural blood clots, 141–44; surgery for, 140–41; vomiting and, 85

headaches: postspinal, 144; and subdural blood clots, 141–42. *See also* migraine headaches
head-tilt maneuver, 107–8
Health Maintenance Organizations (HMO), welfare patients and, 205–6
heart attacks: as cause of death, 5; compared with angina, 20; danger period after, 22; diagnosis of, 12–13, 15–17, 18–22; mistaken for drunkenness, 182–83; paramedics and, 24–30; prevention of deaths from, 13–14; symptoms of, 24. *See also* cardiac arrest
Heimlich maneuver, 108
hematocrit, 93–94; initial, 69–70
hemorrhoids, 101
hemothorax, 57–63, 65–66
hernias, 101
heroin. *See* drug-overdose victims
holding wards, 160
homosexuals, police attitude toward, 173
hymen, broken, 71
hypovolemic shock, 46
hypoxemia, near-drowning and, 115
hypoxia, 121–23

impotence, priapism and, 113
infants: and acute intussusception, 81; artificial ventilation in, 36; swimming reflex in, 114–15
inhalation therapist, xi, xii, 125, 126; and endotracheal intubation, 170; and intermittent positive pressure breathing, 109–10
injuries. *See specific types:* bullet wounds; head injuries, *etc.*
intermittent positive-pressure breathing machine, 109–10
intestinal cancer, 93–94
intestinal obstruction, 81, 82–89
intestine, ruptures of, 78
intraabdominal bleeding, 77–78
intracranial pressure, 85, 121, 122, 127–28
intravenous (IV), xii, 14, 25, 60, 96, 121; in ambulances, 24; in elderly, 39–40; and head injuries, 124; insertion of, 17
intravenous pyelogram, 71–72
intussusception, acute, in infants, 81
Ipecac-induced vomiting, 154–55, 157

kidney damage, 70, 75; diagnosis by intravenous pyelogram, 71–72
kidney pain, 82
kidney stone, diagnosis of, 84

lab tests, 88, 124, 153, 156, 161
large intestine. *See* colon
laws: on suicide attempts, 158–59; on suspected child abuse, 179
life-sustaining machinery, 44
limbo state, 44
litigation: and blood-alcohol tests, 182; and length of cardiopulmonary resuscitation efforts, 44; and minors, 55–56; and skull X-rays, 146; and taped paramedic runs, 25. *See also* malpractice suits
liver injuries, 76–78, 95
lower airway obstructions, 108. *See also* asthma
LSD overdose, 161–66
lung: collapsed, 59–60; salt and fresh water in, 115. *See also* pulmonary edema; pulmonary embolism

malpractice suits, 206–7. *See also* litigation
MAST suit. *See* military antishock trousers
Medicaid, 204–6
medical groups: and "skimmers," 209–10; specializing in welfare patients, 155
menstrual extraction, 193
migraine headaches, 66–67
military antishock trousers, 61–62
Mobile Intensive Care Nurses' Test, 120
Mobile Intensive Care Unit, 3
morning-after pill. *See* DES
morphine, 18, 92
mouth-to-mouth resuscitation, 34–35
multiple injuries, 54–63

nail, removal of, 67
nasogastric tube, 171
nasotracheal intubation, 125–26
nausea, 75. *See also* vomiting
near-drownings, 114–16
neurogenic shock, 47
neurological death, 44
neurosurgeons, brain injuries and, 124, 133, 134, 140–41, 143
nitroglycerine, 18, 19
nurses, 14; and administration of medication and oxygen, 105, 106, 107, 124, 171; and cardiopulmonary resuscitation, 41–42, 44–45, 47; and drug-overdose victims, 153, 155; expectations of, 117–19; and lab tests, 124; and monitor, 183; as patients, 79–81, 83, 89–90; and rape victims, 189; relations with emergency medicine physicians, 104–5, 116–19, 124–25; and suicide attempt victims, 158; and violent patients, 163

objects. *See* foreign objects
oral surgeon, treatment by of bleeding from mouth, 185
otolaryngologist, 136
otoscope, 48–49, 136
oxygen: in ambulance, 24; and asthma, 105; behavior and, 59, 60; and drug-overdose victims, 152. *See also* hypoxia

pain: diagnosis of intraabdominal injury and, 74–75; on left side, 69; PCP and insensitivity to, 162; "real" and "fake," 182; on right side, 76–78; in shoulder, 77–78. *See also* abdominal pain; chest pain
pancreatitis, 81, 82, 85
paracentesis, abdominal bleeding and, 77–78
paramedic calls. *See* biocom calls
paramedics, 3; and cardiopulmonary resuscitation, 33–35; and drug-overdose victims, 149–50; and heart attack victims, 24–26; and medication, 92; role of, 7, 25–26;

and tape reviews, 25; training, 26
parental consent, 55–56
parents: child abusers, 177–80; and injured children, 70–71, 141, 145; and teenage drug use, 161. *See also* families of patients
Parents Anonymous, 178
PCP ("angel dust"), overdoses of, 161–66
Peace Corps, 2
pelvic fractures, bladders and, 75
penicillin, allergy to, 112
penis: injuries to, 22–23, 100; and priapism, 113–14
percussion, abdominal swelling and, 85
Personal Injury System, 207
physician groups, 211
plastic surgeons, 139–40, 180–81
poisoning victims, 154–55, 176–77
police: and accidents, 56; alcoholics and, 95; attitudes toward homosexuals, 173; attitudes toward nurses, 163; attitudes toward patients, 163–65, 167–86; and blood-alcohol tests, 181–82; and child abusers, 177; and gunshot wounds, 147–48; and prebooking exams, 168–69; and rape victims, 188–89
police brutality charges, 173–74
postbooking exam, 168–69
poverty of elderly, 93, 174–76
prebooking exams, 168–69, 173–75, 180–81
pregnancy, rape victims and, 192–93
pregnancy tests, abdominal pain and, 88
priapism, 112–14
pulmonary edema, 47, 115
pulmonary embolism, 25–27
pupils: and brain death, 45; and drug overdoses, xii, 152; and epidural hemorrhage, 123

rabies, 64–65
radiation, and eye injuries, 137
rape, incidence of, 197
rape crisis centers, 197, 199–200
rape victims, 188–201; attitudes toward, 194–95, 197, 200–201; con-

rape victims (*continued*)
   sent form for, 189–90; and DES, 193
rapists, 194–95; "psychiatric" and "criminal," 196–97
rectal examination, 87, 98
rectum, foreign object in, 97–99
referred pain, 78, 82
respiration therapist: and drug overdose victims, 150, 151, 152, 154; and head injuries, 146
rheumatic fever, strep throat and, 111–12
ribs. *See* broken ribs
runaways, 55

"scoop and run" victims, 169–72
Seconal overdose, 153, 154, 155
seizures, 128–30
septic shock, 47
shock, types of, 46–47
shoulder pain, 77–78
Sigmoidoscope, 98
"skimmers," 209–12
skull fractures, 144–46
skull X-rays, 143, 144–47
small intestine, wounds to, 73
sodium bicarbonate, cardiopulmonary resuscitation and, 41, 44
sore throats, 110–12
specialization, 7–8
spinal cord injuries, 47, 170–71
spinal taps, 143–44
spleen, injuries to, 77, 82
sprained ankles, 72–73
stab wounds, 73
stomach: "pumping out," 154–55, 157, 159; swallowed objects in, 48, 49–51. *See also* abdomen
stool, blood in, 93, 95–96
strep throat, 111–12
subdural blood clot, 141–44
sublingual medication, xii
suicide attempts, 146–48, 149–52, 156–60
suturing, 138–40
swimming reflex, 114–15

Thorazine, LSD overdoses and, 163, 164
ticks, 136–37
tongue, and upper-airway obstruction, 36, 106
toxic shock syndrome, 47
tracheostomy, 125–26
transfusions, 60–61. *See also* blood typing and crossmatching

ulcer, intestinal, 96. *See also* gastric ulcer
ultraviolet rays, eye injuries from, 137
unconsciousness, 125, 150
upper airway obstruction, 106, 107–8
urinary output, 45–46
urination difficulties, 127, 128, 131
urine, blood in, 70, 75
urologists, 113, 116

Valium: and LSD overdose, 162; overdose of, 156–60
venereal disease, rape victims and, 191, 192
venous cutdown, 40
ventricular fibrillation, 183
violent patients, 169–74
vital signs, 16, 17, 24. *See also* blood pressure
vomiting: blood, 95; and cardiac arrest, 37, 38; and diagnosis of abdominal pain, 85–86; induced, 154–55, 177; and intestinal obstruction, 85; seizures and, 129–30; unexpected pregnancy and, 88

welfare patients, 155, 203–7
wet lung. *See* pulmonary edema
wheezing: asthma and, 109; congestive heart failure and, 187–88

X-rays: of bladder, 75; ordered by athletic coaches, 72–73. *See also* intravenous pyelogram *and under individual types:* chest X-rays, skull X-rays, *etc.*